Nursing Support for Families of Dying Patients

Nursing Support for Families of Dying Patients

ROSEMARY MCINTYRE PHD, MN, RGN,
DIPN(LONDON), NDN(CERT), RNT

*Head of Studies (Scotland and Northern Ireland),
Marie Curie Cancer Care (Education)*

W
WHURR PUBLISHERS
LONDON AND PHILADELPHIA

© 2002 Whurr Publishers Ltd
First published 2002
by Whurr Publishers Ltd
19b Compton Terrace
London N1 2UN England and
325 Chestnut Street, Philadelphia PA 19106 USA

Reprinted 2002 and 2005

British Library Cataloguing in Publication Data

A catalogue record for this book
is available from the British Library.

ISBN 1 86156 270 5

Contents

Foreword

The challenges involved in nursing dying patients are widely recognised and have been well researched. However the role of the nurse in supporting the dying patient's family has been given relatively little attention. Rosemary McIntyre's book is therefore particularly welcome and an important contribution to our understanding of this field. The motivation for the study sprang from her awareness of the problems faced by both nurses and relatives in communicating with one another at a time of great anxiety and stress. These problems are clearly delineated in the early part of the book and highlight the fact that nurses have a tendency to avoid prolonged contact because they are uncertain how to respond to the distress of the family. For their part, family members perceive the nurses to be very busy and, accordingly, feel inhibited about approaching them.

The research study that Rosemary McIntyre developed as a result of these problems was inspirational to all those who were involved with it. She saw that there was a need to 'build a bridge' between nurses and relatives and that this could be achieved through a series of carefully planned study 'phases' that included investigation, intervention and evaluation. The theory and methods that form the foundation for such a piece of work are crucial to its success and these are comprehensively described and explained. As the study progressed, a number of conflicts arose as a result of the tension between trying to sustain the role of an objective researcher and having to adopt the role of active participant in the process of 'designing' and 'building the bridge'. Rosemary McIntyre reports these methodological challenges candidly and offers a meticulous account of how she addressed them.

The findings that emerged from the study are illustrated throughout the book with quotations from the participants that are both poignant and illuminating. They make the book required reading for all nursing staff involved in supporting the relatives of dying patients. Of equal importance are the central messages that emerge from the study about the communication and support strategies that nurses can develop in the ward situation. It is a tribute not only to Rosemary McIntyre, but also to the staff nurse participants in the study, that 'the bridge' was successfully built. While the effort involved in a sustained, research-based practice development on this scale should not be under-estimated, this study shows that nurses can overcome barriers to communication at a number of different levels and make a significant contribution to supporting relatives at a time of great distress.

This book is a valuable resource for a number of different audiences. Firstly, for both experienced and inexperienced researchers who are conducting empirical work in the healthcare field, it provides insight into a number of key methodological challenges and how these may be addressed. It also offers an exemplar for those undertaking qualitative analysis. Details of process and issues of rigour are presented critically but in an accessible way. Secondly, the book provides unique material for those involved in the education of nurses at pre- and post-registration levels. The quotations from nurses and relatives and the paradigm cases in Chapter 9 could be used illustratively in teaching sessions or as a basis for discussion in small groups. Finally nurses and other health care professionals involved in supporting relatives of the dying patient cannot fail to benefit from this book. Rosemary McIntyre has opened a window onto some very testing personal and professional experiences that bring to life the dilemmas faced by relatives and nurses. She also shows how nurses responded to these dilemmas and developed a range of approaches to support their practice. It is vital that these receive critical attention and that they are further evaluated in practice.

Jean McIntosh
Glasgow Caledonian University
October 2001

Preface

My interest in family support during terminal illness stems from my own clinical nursing background. As a District Nurse I noted that the context of community care seemed to support more readily a family focused approach to terminal care, presumably because the care setting avoids separation of the dying patient from their close family and from their home environment. When I was caring for dying patients in hospital, however, bringing relatives into the focus of care always seemed to me to be particularly challenging. Following a patient's death in hospital, nurses often reported having been left with the uncomfortable feeling that more could, and indeed should, have been done for the family of a particular patient who had died. Later, when I was a nurse educator, students continued to offer convincing evidence that the extended presence of dying patients' relatives causes difficulties for staff who are unsure how best to meet the needs of these 'non patients' who are in and around the hospital ward.

It was from this background that the following questions emerged:

- When relatives stay for extended periods around the ward with their dying loved one, what is it that they need from the staff?
- What are the factors that make this aspect of care so challenging for nurses?
- How might staff be enabled to meet the needs of these families with less discomfort to themselves?

In seeking answers to these questions I felt it important to explore the perspectives of both the relatives and the nurses. By seeking this dual perspective I hoped that specific aspects of the interface between the family and staff might be illuminated. Moreover, while this study was conducted within an academic framework and led to the award of PhD, I had the firm wish to avoid the common situation where researchers seek out shortfalls in practice and then simply report these deficiencies. I wanted to try to take the next step and to explore, with the practitioners, what, if anything, they felt could be done to address issues that might emerge. To accommodate this an intervention study was planned. It was felt that this approach would best support the development, implementation and evaluation of any interventions that the practitioners had determined were necessary. Crucially these interventions would be informed by the data obtained from interviews with relatives and nurses from the study wards during the first phase of the study.

Throughout the course of the study I worked with a remarkable team of 16 Staff Nurses drawn from eight acute wards in two major city hospitals in Scotland. Together the nurses and I formed the 'research team', and there is no doubt at all that without their cooperation and commitment the work quite simply could not have been done. Each of the nurses participated in a pre-intervention and in a post-intervention interview. Data derived from these interviews offered valuable insights into the professional carer's perspective on family care during very advanced illness. The nurses also assisted with recruitment of the relatives' samples required for pre- and post-intervention interviews.

During the extended intervention period the nurses worked very actively within their own wards to bring about changes in practice which they, and their colleagues on the ward, had agreed were required. At the end of this book there is one example of a Quality Assurance Standard and audit tool produced at ward level. In reality eight quite separate standards were developed and the emphasis and content of each differed slightly to reflect locally defined priorities within each ward.

In fulfilling this demanding role many of the nurses were very fortunate to have the support and commitment of managers and peers. One or two were less fortunate and they had to work very creatively to bring about changes in a climate of resistance and apathy. Overall, and to the great credit of the nurses in the research team, the positive changes in practice that were achieved were considerable.

Working with this team of nurses was an experience for which I am grateful. They brought an immense energy to the research work but they also ensured that I remained firmly grounded in the real, practical and fascinating world of clinical practice. With those nurses in mind I now offer this work, hopefully as an accessible account of a collaborative effort where researcher and practitioners worked together for the common goal of improving care and support for relatives of dying patients.

While the work focused on relatives of *cancer* patients, this diagnostic distinction was made on methodological grounds alone. Insights gained, and interventions developed, from this work are applicable right across the spectrum of illnesses and indeed across different care settings. Indeed I hope that the findings will have resonance with staff who are providing care for patients who are dying from whatever cause. By subtle shifts in attitudes, and by relatively simple changes in practice, the study showed that relatives can be brought out of the shadows into the focus of care.

Acknowledgements

Grateful thanks are extended to every relative who participated in this study and who did so while in the throes of dealing with the imminent loss of a loved one. The relatives' generosity in sharing their feelings and experiences during this difficult time has provided insights that could illuminate the way for nurses to improve the quality of support offered to the dying patient's family in hospital. Sincere appreciation is also extended to the participating staff nurses who worked with such energy, commitment and sensitivity to improve care for relatives of dying patients and to motivate their colleagues to work with them on this initiative. The clarity and honesty with which they shared their concerns and feelings during their interviews vividly revealed the costs and the rewards that can come from caring.

I would also like to thank Miss CA Asher (OBE), Acting Principal, Glasgow College of Nursing and Midwifery (retired) who provided much encouragement and support for this work and who, together with Professor Margaret Alexander of the Department of Nursing and Community Health in Glasgow Caledonian University, was instrumental in getting this study launched. Subsequent funding for the main study came in the form of a Nursing Research Fellowship from the Greater Glasgow Health Board. The support provided by the Health Board, and in particular from Mrs B Maclennan (Acting Chief Area Nursing Officer) is gratefully acknowledged. The cooperation of the Directors of Nursing Services and their Senior Nurse Managers, Quality Assurance Nurses and staff in the study wards has also been appreciated.

The contribution of the workshop facilitators, Jean Kellet and Liz McConnell, is also gratefully acknowledged. The energy and enthusiasm that they generated at the workshop provided a vital driving force for the staff nurses as they set about the difficult process of implementing changes in their practice area.

Academic supervision has been provided by Professor Jean McIntosh and Professor Margaret Alexander. I feel privileged to have been guided by these nursing scholars. In particular, I will always be grateful to Jean McIntosh, my Director of Studies, whose support, guidance and unflagging belief in this research work have sustained me through some challenging times when my confidence might otherwise have faltered.

Research is often viewed as a somewhat solitary enterprise. I am glad to say that has not been my experience. The camaraderie of the staff in the Department of Nursing and Community Health in Glasgow Caledonian University and the friendship of my research colleagues have been appreciated and enjoyed. Philip Darbyshire offered a challenging and encouraging sounding board for my developing insights into hermeneutics and Christina Knussen, from the Department of Psychology, helped me explore links between coping theory and the emerging data. Thanks are also offered to Marian Miller, the Faculty Librarian, for professional assistance and advice.

Finally, challenges always seem less daunting when we feel the support of caring people around us. This has been especially important in a study such as this that has contained so much grief and sadness. My husband, family and my very good friends have all ensured that I kept a healthy perspective that has focused on living, and loving and laughing.

Quotation

May there never develop in me the notion that my education is complete, but give me strength and licence and zeal continually to enlarge my knowledge.

Maimonides – daily prayer of a physician

Chapter 1
Introduction

When a patient has advanced cancer, considerable demands are placed on the whole family. While coping with their own profound emotions, close relatives commonly have to support their loved ones through a range of treatments as the disease progresses through stages of remission and recurrence until, finally, a shift to a palliative mode of treatment must be faced. In such situations, family roles and relationships are likely to be disrupted and family members' coping resources can be stretched to the limit. It is clear from this that, by the time the terminal stage of the patient's illness is reached, the family may have travelled a long and difficult road, and close relatives are likely to be emotionally vulnerable and in need of support.

The researcher's own nursing experience with dying patients and their families, in both hospital and community settings, and her experience as a volunteer with a cancer support group, offered persuasive, albeit anecdotal, evidence that close relatives of dying patients often have unmet needs for support. Impressions from both care settings seemed to suggest that, within the complex structures of hospitals, where the number and range of patients and professional carers are greater, supporting the dying patient's family presents particular difficulties for staff.

Undoubtedly, it can also be painful and demanding for health professionals to be regularly confronted with death and faced with the grief of others. The researcher's experience in nurse education highlighted some issues that concern nursing students as they approach the end of their pre-registration education. Although students commonly report a degree of anxiety about their future role as staff nurses, a recurrent concern frequently voiced by students relates to how they should deal with the dying patient's family around the time of death.

These impressions, coming from a range of different sources, raised a number of interrelated issues. It seemed clear that those who provide care in hospital need to know more about what relatives of dying patients require from nursing staff. It was therefore judged to be important to obtain the relatives' perspective on how staff might better support them during this difficult time.

Reflection on the professional carer's perspective raised other questions. There also seemed to be a need to identify those factors that make support of the dying patient's family stressful for nurses and to establish the support that is needed to enable staff to care for the terminally ill patient's family with less distress to themselves.

This study addresses these fundamental issues using qualitative research approaches, which should allow the salient issues to be explored from both the relatives' and the nurses' perspectives, and should also enable a research-based intervention, aimed at improving family care and support, to be designed, implemented and evaluated.

Structure of the book

In Chapter 2, the literature is reported in four main sections, including the context within which terminal care for cancer patients is provided, the relatives' perspective on care provision, communication issues within the hospital setting and the professional carers' perspective on this aspect of their role. The literature clearly confirms that provision of care and support for the dying patient's family in the acute hospital setting is indeed problematic for both relatives and nurses.

Chapter 3 presents the choice of theoretical framework for the study. A 'cognitive, phenomenological, transactional model', based on Lazarus's theory of stress and coping (Wrubel, Benner and Lazarus 1981), was selected for the study. This framework was favoured mainly because stress emerged as an all-pervasive theme in the literature and also because this particular model recognizes the unique, subjective nature of each participant's experiences and feelings.

Chapter 4 describes and supports the choice of research method. The dynamic and evolving character of the study design is revealed as the sampling methods, interview approach and analysis techniques are described. In Chapter 5 findings from the relatives' and the nurses' phase 1 analysis are presented. In each case, the data are organized and reported in themes. Presentation and discussion of these themes parallel the approach, volume and depth of the feedback provided for the staff nurses at the start of the 2-day workshop, which formed part of the intervention.

Chapter 6 provides an account of the intervention: the aims, structure and conduct of the workshop, and the processes involved in the development, implementation and evaluation of quality assurance standards for improved family support during terminal illness. The complex processes involved in implementing a planned change initiative over a range of clinical settings are described with reference to the literature on action research and change theory.

Chapter 7 reports the results of the relatives' phase 2 (post-intervention) analysis and in Chapter 8 the nurses' phase 2 findings are similarly reported. The comparative analysis approach used in these chapters, together with additional evaluation data presented in Chapter 9, provides the framework for evaluating the impact of the intervention.

Chapter 10 considers the extent to which the aims and objectives of the study have been met and the implications of the research findings for nursing practice discussed. In this final chapter, limitations of the study are acknowledged and conclusions and recommendations offered.

Chapter 2
Review of the literature

The initial search of the literature was directed at establishing current knowledge about the experience of terminal illness from the dual perspectives of the dying patient's family and the nurses who provide care in hospital wards. Evidence gleaned from the literature informed the design of the study and the research instruments. As the study evolved, the reviewing processes developed a cyclical character as it became clear that additional areas such as change theory, action research and quality assurance needed to be revised. Also, new channels of enquiry opened up as the researcher sought deeper understanding of the complex issues that were emerging from analysis of the nurses' and relatives' interview data. The result has been a wide-ranging and ongoing engagement with the literature, some sections of which is reported elsewhere. Literature relating to theories of stress and coping is reported in Chapter 3. The research methods and ethics literature are included in Chapter 4, and theories underpinning planned change inform discussions on the intervention in Chapter 6.

The literature that is reported in this chapter has been organized into four main sections, each of which contains a number of key themes.

The first section explores the context of terminal illness. Evidence that cancer remains a major cause of death in Scotland and that caring for patients with advanced cancer and supporting the dying patient's family are still significant aspects of care in the hospital setting are examined. A brief review of developments in the provision of care for patients with advanced cancer is also undertaken.

In the second section, the literature focuses on the relatives' experiences, and the stresses and the demands associated with having a close relative who has advanced cancer. Sources that explore the effects of advanced disease on family roles and relationships and identify the coping strategies employed by relatives are reported. In particular, works that explore strategies such as avoidance, denial and hope are reviewed.

The third section represents a major section of the review. It was judged important to uncover literature that highlights the needs of relatives during the terminal stages of the patient's illness, and the ways in which nurses can best meet these needs. Literature that reports significant unmet needs for communication and information is reported and a literature-based analysis of the factors that influence communication between relatives and staff within the hospital setting offered.

The fourth section focuses on the experiences of health-care personnel. Particular attention is directed at literature that explores the nature and extent of stress engendered in nursing staff by caring for the dying patient's family, and the coping strategies that nurses employ. Finally, literature-based evidence about the roots, consequences and prevention of the phenomenon of 'burnout' in nurses is briefly reported.

The context

Epidemiology

International statistical sources reveal that Scotland ranks top for lung cancer deaths and is second from the top in overall female cancer mortality (Muir and Harvey 1994). Scottish statistical data confirm that deaths from cancer represent around 25% of all deaths in Scotland (Registrar General for Scotland 1994; Greater Glasgow Health Board 1995).

Table 2.1 presents the Scottish cancer mortality figures for 1994 and confirms that most cancer-related deaths occurred in hospital. It also reveals that dealing with dying patients remains a common experience for certain groups of hospital nurses. Furthermore, over the past three decades changes in demographic and disease patterns, and a shift from acute to chronic illness as a cause of death, have led

Table 2.1: Number and place of cancer deaths in Scotland

All places	Home	NHS hospital	Non-NHS hospital/ hospice	Homes for elderly and disabled people	Other homes
15 458	4045	9774	1507	129	3
Percentage of total	26.17	63.23	9.75	0.83	0.02

Registrar General for Scotland (1994).

to a steady growth in the demand for provision of palliative care services (Higginson 1993; Seale 1993; Eve and Jackson 1994; Ford 1994). The nature and scope of this care provision are briefly considered below and the terminology defined.

Palliative care provision

Palliative care represents the active total care of patients for whom curative treatment is no longer possible and for whom control of physical, psychological, social and spiritual problems is paramount. Effective palliative care should provide a support system to enable patients to live as actively as possible until death and should help the family cope during the patient's illness and with their bereavement (World Health Organization 1990). Terminal care refers to the care that is given during the very late stages of the illness, where there is a steady deterioration in the patient's condition and death is judged to be close (Scottish Partnership Agency for Palliative and Cancer Care 1995).

Although most patients who receive palliative care have a primary diagnosis of cancer, increasingly it is being recognized that the principles of palliative care can be applied to the care of people with other chronic progressive diseases (Doyle 1984; Harris 1990; Marks 1992). The development of specialist care in the UK can be traced to the 1960s, when a number of authors highlighted severe shortcomings in institutional care for dying patients (Glaser and Strauss 1965; Sudnow 1967). In response to these reported deficiencies, Cicely Saunders developed an approach to care that emphasized symptom control, psychosocial support and more open communication about death, which was to become the hallmark of future hospice care (Seale 1989).

There is now a growing recognition of the need to extend the philosophy and principles of palliative care, laid down by Saunders, into community and hospital settings where most patients still die (Dicks 1990; Anstey 1993; Webber 1993) (Table 2.1). To this end, hospital and community staff are increasingly able to access advice and support from symptom control teams and specialist home care teams (Seale 1989; Scottish Partnership Agency for Palliative and Cancer Care 1995). Developments in palliative care provision have been accompanied by a growing body of research and by a range of specialist journals and professional associations (Corner 1991a; Franks and Ahmedzai 1995; Jackson 1995).

Nursing developments in this area were spearheaded by organizations such as Cancer Relief Macmillan and Marie Curie Cancer Care which provide support, counselling and home nursing services. More recently, an increasing number of nurse specialists have been appointed in hospitals, hospices or regional cancer centres to provide specific nursing expertise and to enhance the continuity of care among hospital, hospice and community settings (Scottish Partnership Agency for Palliative and Cancer Care 1995).

Table 2.1 confirms that, although most patients die in hospital, they may have received care in other settings during the course of their illness. To understand patients' and relatives' experiences of different contexts of care, these are briefly reviewed.

The care settings

As the focus of the current study is on terminal care within the hospital setting, only a very brief review of hospice or home-care studies is offered. This literature is included in recognition of the fact that relatives in the current study might have experienced care for their loved one in home and/or hospice settings before the final admission, and this could colour their current perceptions of hospital care.

Care in the home

Cartwright, in a replication of an earlier study conducted in 1969 into life and care during the last year of life, found that 81% of the deceased patients had spent most of the last year of their lives in their own homes (Cartwright, Hockey and Anderson 1973; Cartwright 1991). Other findings from this later study revealed that more dying people now live alone or with a spouse only, when compared with 1969, and more of the people studied were over 75 years of age. These findings have clear implications for family caregivers.

Stetz interviewed 65 spouses of cancer patients whose disease was at various stages and who were being cared for at home (Stetz 1987). The most pressing demands reported by these caregivers related to difficulties encountered managing the patient's physical care (69%), the distress associated with witnessing the patient's deterioration (39%), and managing household, social and financial matters (39%) (Stetz 1987). Stetz conducted a 6-month follow-up interview with 31 bereaved spouses from the original sample of 65. More than half of the second sample expressed regrets about their care-giving efforts and reported that they wished they had sought out and used more resources. To reduce future regret, Stetz recommends that care staff should assist relatives to recognize their needs for outside help and support during the demanding care-giving period (Stetz and Hanson 1992).

When interpreting these findings, it should be noted that 53% ($n = 34$) of the original sample either declined a second interview or could not be traced. However, other studies corroborate Stetz's findings, consistently highlighting the physical and emotional demands associated with care-giving and indicating significant unmet needs for support (Hinds 1985; Herity et al. 1987; Lewandowski and Jones 1988; Hull 1989a; Hunt 1991a). These authors consistently report significant caregiver stress. In particular, findings from Hull's (1990) study, which used ethnographic techniques to study relatives in an American hospice–home care programme, revealed a complex array of stresses associated with the caregiver role, often requiring the relative to relinquish this role and to seek hospital admission before the patient's death. Hull's sample was small ($n = 14$) and heterogeneous in terms of age and relationship to the patient. However, the relatives were interviewed monthly throughout their care-giving experience with a final interview one month after the patient's death; the numbers of interviews per family ranged from two to ten (Hull 1989a). It should also be noted that hospice care within the USA health-care context usually refers to an outpatient or day-care facility.

In a major UK survey, a questionnaire-and-interview approach was used, with a sample of 65 terminally ill cancer patients and their family carers, to investigate their current problems and needs and to elicit their views about care provision (Higginson, Wade and McCarty 1990). Stress on the main carer and problems experienced in achieving adequate symptom control were the most frequently reported problems by both patients and carers (Higginson et al. 1990). High levels of caregiver anxiety and difficulties associated with symptom control have been consistently reported in the literature (Higginson et al. 1990; Kristjanson and Ashcroft 1994). Indeed, these authors concur that relatives' needs often exceed those of the dying patients and need to be separately assessed.

Parkes (1988) compared symptom control and psychosocial support in home or hospital/hospice care. Findings indicate that, in the home-care context, the time between stopping active treatment and death was more than three times longer than in hospital; symptom control was reported as less effective and the degree of family strain was significantly higher (Parkes 1988). Terminal care in the home was often associated with significant suffering for both patients and relatives. Parkes' findings also suggest that the final days of the patient's illness were more emotionally intense and distressing for the family than for the patient. Parkes, and a number of other authors, suggest that subsequent grief reactions may be influenced by such factors as the duration and location of the death, and the effectiveness of symptom control (Parkes 1988; Kristjanson 1989; Klagsbrun 1994).

Having noted the difficulties that many care-giving relatives encounter within the home-care setting, the next section reviews the literature that relates to the hospice and hospital setting.

Care in the hospice and hospital setting

There is a dearth of evidence in the literature to support claims that hospice care is superior to conventional care. Indeed, Seale (1989) claims that in the UK little is currently known about the ways in which hospices differ from each other or about how hospitals and hospices differ. In the course of his study, Seale interviewed relatives of 45 cancer patients dying in a hospice setting and relatives of 126 dying cancer patients receiving conventional care either in hospital or at home. The author concluded that it has yet to be firmly established that hospice staff practise a distinctive approach to care. To advance understanding of how palliative care settings differ, and to clarify some of the existing ideological debates, studies of patient, staff and relative communications within different care settings are recommended as are interview studies to explore relatives' judgements about the care experienced in different care settings (Seale 1989).

To explore satisfaction with care provision around the time of death, an interview study was conducted with 51 bereaved relatives of patients who had died in hospital or hospice settings in the UK (Bolton Health Council 1986). Although many patients had received care in more than one setting, all had spent some time in hospital and most had experienced terminal care there. Relatives' judgements about hospital care were mixed. Although some praised the nursing care highly, others reported that staff were sometimes unhelpful or 'too busy' to deal with them. Gaining access to staff, and to information about the patient, also proved to be very stressful for relatives (Bolton Health Council 1986). This finding, that relatives experience difficulty in accessing information in the hospital setting, is widely corroborated elsewhere (Maguire and Faulkner 1988; Kristjanson 1989; Higginson et al. 1990).

The authors of the Bolton survey conclude that hospitals urgently need to improve their arrangements for dealing with visitors of seriously ill patients. They assert that little thought appears to have been given to relatives' needs, and that facilities for the comfort and privacy of the dying patient's close family in hospital were patchy or inadequate. Few had access to a visitors' room, although in many wards nurses did supply easy chairs and blankets, which were appreciated by the relatives (Bolton Health Council 1986). Satisfaction with hospice care was high, although some relatives found the hospice environment difficult to cope with (Bolton Health Council 1986). Although now some 10 years old, these findings remain pertinent to the current study. Also, in the light of recent interest in quality assurance in health care, and in keeping with the spirit of the Patient's Charter (Scottish Office 1991), this is an area that merits investigation.

Higginson et al. (1990) sought the judgements of 65 dying cancer patients and their main carer ($n = 65$) about different forms of care that they had received. The relatives' judgements about the quality of different forms of care provision are summarized below (Higginson et al. 1990).

Relatives' ratings of care provision

> Specialist support teams were rated 'good' or 'excellent' by 89% of patients and by 91% of relatives.
>
> General practitioners and district nurses were rated 'good' or 'excellent' by 71% of patients and 71% of relatives.
>
> Hospital doctors and nurses were rated 'good' or 'excellent' by 34% of patients and 54% of relatives.
>
> (Higginson et al. 1990)

In this study, the relatives' most frequently reported difficulties focused on poor communication in hospital, poorly coordinated services, hospital doctors' 'attitudes', in that senior medical staff at times appeared distant and superior in their manner, and perceived delays in reaching a diagnosis (Higginson et al. 1990). When interpreting these findings, however, it should be noted that the palliative care support team, who were the most positively evaluated care providers, were themselves responsible for referring families who were currently under their care into the study. Moreover, patients who required to be referred for specialist support might well have had unresolved difficulties while under the care of the primary care team or hospital staff, which could have coloured their judgements of these care providers. While acknowledging these potential areas of bias, there is nonetheless ample corroborating evidence of the low level of satisfaction that families expressed with terminal care within the hospital setting (Herity et al. 1987; Faulkner 1988a; Fallowfield 1993a). In particular, Fallowfield (1993a) comments on the insensitive treatment that patients and relatives report within the hospital setting, especially in relation to communication about the patient's prognosis (Fallowfield 1993a).

The Health Service Commissioner's report on the quality of care provided for dying patients and their families in NHS hospitals in England provided the impetus for a survey to elicit relatives' views about the care that had been provided around the time of their loved one's death (Wright, Cousins and Upward 1988). A radio station launched the study and invited comments from recently bereaved relatives whose loved one had died in hospital. Contact with the researchers was by using a special telephone line or by letter. Of the 119 telephone calls received, only 25 were judged to be 'positive'

(Wright et al. 1988). The relatives' main reported concerns related to unsympathetic attitudes of staff, problems with communication, difficulties gaining access to information, and lack of support for the family around the time of the death. The authors of this survey conclude that 'the scope for improving care for dying patients and their families in hospital is enormous' (Wright et al. 1988).

Some caution should be exercised when interpreting these findings because sampling relied on self-referral of relatives and data gathering was mainly by telephone interview. It is also possible that those relatives who were dissatisfied with the care received might have been most highly motivated to respond. Despite these potential limitations the findings of this survey are well supported elsewhere (Bolton Health Council 1986; Hempel 1988; Health Service Commissioner for England, Scotland and Wales 1995).

Relatives' judgements about care in hospital can also be influenced by a number of factors, e.g. the speed at which the illness progresses will affect the family's responses and coping strategies and, in situations where there is a steep downward trajectory, interactions with staff tend to be brief. In such situations, relatives may receive inadequate information and have less time to prepare for the death (Kristjanson and Ashcroft 1994). Conversely, a lingering, prolonged vigil has been found to engender feelings of guilt as relatives wait for the death to occur (Kristjanson and Ashcroft 1994).

This section of the literature has established that the numbers of people who experience cancer within their close family circle are considerable and that caring for dying cancer patients and their families remains a significant aspect of hospital practice. It has also been established that the needs of relatives are not always adequately met within the hospital setting. It follows from this that staff who provide terminal care in hospital might benefit from hearing the relatives' perspective on how terminal illness is experienced within the family.

The relatives' perspective

Family stress

Health professionals are now coming to recognize that cancer is experienced not just by the patient but by the entire family (Hull 1989a; Woods et al. 1989; Kristjanson and Ashcroft 1994). Although the experiences of each family, and indeed of each family member, will be unique, there are a number of common factors that influence their experiences during the terminal illness (Northouse and Northouse 1987; Woods et al. 1989). As the family usually represents the patient's primary source of support, it was judged necessary to reflect briefly on literature that explores how the family unit, and the behaviour and responses of individual family members, might be affected by a life-threatening illness.

There is now a growing literature that focuses on family functioning within the context of serious illness. Davies, writing on her own and with others (Davies 1990; Davies and Oberle 1990; Davies, Reimer and Martens 1994), analysed data from a series of qualitative studies conducted in Canada to explore family functioning during terminal illness. The authors conclude that the entire family should be the focus of care during terminal illness, and they recommend that nurses need to adjust their interventions to recognize the disruptive effects of illness on family functioning and to support the integrity of the family unit (Davies et al. 1994). These authors developed an approach to assessment based on various dimensions of family functioning (Davies et al. 1994). In one study they used grounded theory method, with a sample of 24 family members drawn from eight families with a dying member (Davies 1990). Findings reveal the dynamic character of the relatives' experiences, which Davies describes in terms of a series of transitions. In particular the very advanced stage was reported as all pervading in character and highly demanding emotionally (Davies 1990).

Although overall patterns of family coping during a fatal illness are poorly understood, it has been mooted that a family's habitual coping style, such as assertion or powerlessness in the face of stress or challenge, might also be manifested during the terminal illness (Davies et al. 1994). These findings are supported by a number of other authors who report that the effects of cancer on family functioning will vary with the stage of the disease, the developmental stage of the family, and the accepted roles and relationships that operate within the family (Cooper 1984; Wilson and Morse 1991).

During a progressive illness, shifts and negotiations in family roles occur in response to changes in the patient's condition, and difficulties can be encountered as the family tries to respond to fluctuating and often subtle changes in the ill person's condition (Kristjanson and Ashcroft 1994). The fluidity and adaptation of family roles during a fatal illness involve hard work and negotiation on the part of the family, often resulting in significant stress (Holmes and Rahe 1967; Kristjanson and Ashcroft 1994). Families found to adapt best were those with older children who could cope with expanded roles and those in which there had been good spousal communication before the illness (Kristjanson and Ashcroft 1994).

These findings have relevance to nurses when they are assessing the support needs of close family members. Of particular interest is the large number of female caregivers who simultaneously face the demands of ageing parents and those of their own children (Kristjanson and Ashcroft 1994). Such women can experience multiple stresses and emotional conflicts as they endeavour to respond to the array of demands that are placed on them (Nugent 1988; Kristjanson and Ashcroft 1994). Societal expectations that female relatives will function as primary caregivers was confirmed by Johnson, who found that 73% of primary caregivers of dying patients were female relatives and a further 5% were significantly involved in the provision of care (Johnson, Cockburn and Pegler 1988). Although these (mainly female) caregivers bear a considerable physical and emotional burden, and often experience health problems attributable to the stress of caring, their support needs go largely unrecognized (Nugent 1988). Hull (1989a, 1990) similarly argues that little attention has been directed at establishing how these relatives cope with the demands placed on them.

In Hull's doctoral research, reported in the first section of this review, 14 family caregivers were interviewed monthly throughout the course of the care-giving experience with a final follow-up interview 3 weeks after the patient's death (Hull 1989a). Findings reveal a number of phases in the family cancer experience, the first of which involves 'confronting reality'. At this point, the family are brought to recognize the terminal nature of their loved one's illness. Faced with the inevitability of their loved one's death, relatives move to the stage of 'surveying the options' for care. A period of 'immersion' follows during which the relative disengages from other responsibilities to focus exclusively on the caring role. At this stage care-giving is an all-pervading concern; an array of stressors are experienced by the carer and a range of coping strategies employed. 'Re-focusing' is the final phase where often, for a variety of reasons, relatives have to relinquish the care-giving role and re-focus on alternative approaches to care for their loved one, such as hospital care (Hull 1989a).

Within the hospital setting, female relatives frequently function as the main point of contact between the family and the staff. Moreover, many will have been the patient's main caregiver at home and will be dealing with the emotional repercussion of the final admission. Hull (1989a) urges further investigation into the emotional consequences for caregivers of either continuing with, or having to relinquish, the caregiver role (Hull 1989a). Hull's sample was small in that she studied only 10 families ($n = 14$). However, a total of 55 interviews was conducted and the resulting transcripts were subjected to content analysis. The strength of this study lies in the repeated interviews which enabled the relatives' experiences to be explored over a period of time, thus acknowledging, and revealing, the dynamic character of the family experience of terminal illness.

Terminal illness has been revealed as a stress experience of such pervasiveness that it can severely tax the coping resources of the close family. The extent of this suffering is increasingly being acknowledged because it affects not just the patient but also the family and in particular the primary caregiver (Nugent, 1988; Davies and Oberle 1990; Herth 1993; Gregory and English 1994; Klagsbrun 1994). Having to stand by and witness the physical, and sometimes also the mental, deterioration in the condition of a loved one has been judged to be the most stressful aspect of the experience for close relatives (Stetz and Hanson 1992).

Distress of this magnitude has significant implications for care. The literature offers substantial confirmation of the social isolation and lack of support that many relatives and family caregivers experience during their loved one's final illness (Kirschling 1986; Kristjanson 1986; Matson 1988; Jones 1991; Houston and Kendall 1992).

Support needs of relatives

A review of the literature that reported relatives' judgements about nursing interventions experienced during their loved one's terminal illness revealed the most highly valued nursing behaviours to be those geared towards providing relatives with regular information and promoting the patient's physical comfort. Interventions directed at meeting the family's own needs were consistently rated less important than patient-focused activities (Hull 1989a). In the hospital setting, relatives reported the need to remain in close proximity to their loved one, and they reported anxiety if the accommodation they were given was at a distance from the patient's bedside (Hull 1989a).

Literature reporting the support for the dying patient's family in hospitals consistently reveals that the relatives' most pressing needs are for regular information about their loved one's care and treatment, and for assurances of the patient's comfort and freedom from distressing symptoms (Hinds 1985; Wright et al. 1988). These findings are corroborated in the results of a Q Sort administered to 20 relatives of dying cancer patients (Skorupka and Bohnet 1982). Behaviours judged by relatives as most supportive were those directed at keeping the patient comfortable, keeping the family fully informed and conveying the nurses' availability (Skorupka and Bohnet 1982). It should, however, be noted that the Q Sort items in Skorupka's study were generated by 'expert nurses' rather than family members, which might influence judgements about validity.

Kristjanson used family generated items in a Q Sort as part of a three-stage project to develop and test a tool to measure family satisfaction with terminal care in different care settings (Kristjanson 1986, 1989, 1993). In phase 1, qualitative methods were used to generate indicators of family satisfaction with care. In phase 2 a Q Sort of these items was administered to 210 family members. Cluster analysis reduced these to the 20 most salient indicators of satisfaction with care and support, of which five of the seven top ranked items were found to relate to communication. Relatives' most pressing support needs included the following: to be assured of the patient's comfort, to be given regular information about the patient's condition and to be assured of the availability of a hospital bed. These findings confirm those of Hull (1989a) that patient-focused nursing interventions were consistently ranked higher than those directed at meeting the family's needs (Kristjanson 1989).

Relatives' seemingly low expectations of having their own support needs met have been widely reported elsewhere (Hampe 1975; Hockley 1989; Hull 1989a).

Relatives have reported intense feelings of helplessness, isolation and distress during the patient's terminal illness, together with the perception of having received little support from health professionals or others (Oberst, Thomas and Ward 1989). Such unmet support needs in relatives were also reported by Northouse and Northouse (1987), who found that, although spouses of patients with breast cancer experienced as much (or more) emotional distress as the patients, they received little support. The social isolation and distress that close relatives can experience during the advanced stages of the patient's illness have now been widely reported (Matson 1988; Nugent 1988; Davies et al. 1994; Klagsbrun 1994). In the light of this convincing evidence, Nugent (1988) argues that nurses need to be sensitive to the plight of the dying patient's family, and to their needs for supportive interventions and access to appropriate referral systems.

Nugent (1988) studied the social support needs of 24 family caregivers of dying patients at home. To elicit the relatives' support needs, Nugent (1988) used an 11-item questionnaire interview and an adapted version of the Norbeck Social Support Questionnaire (NSSQ) (Norbeck 1986). Nugent (1988) found that around half of the care-giving relatives lived alone with their dying loved one, and their support needs included the presence of supportive others such as friends, family and health professionals, the timely mobilization of services and resources to support their care-giving efforts, and opportunities for periods of 'time out'. Limitations of this study mainly relate to the small sample and to the limited provision for indepth responses which the data-gathering method offered.

A synthesis of the literature that reports the support needs of relatives of *hospitalized* dying patients reveals that, within the hospital setting, relatives feel supported when they can see the same nurse regularly and when they are given regular information about the patient's condition and care (Kristjanson 1986; Northouse and Northouse 1987; Hockley 1989; Hull 1989a; Davies and Oberle 1990).

Relatives' coping responses

The ways in which families cope with terminal illness are still poorly understood, but it is likely that the main coping strategies employed will be directed primarily at trying to manage the distressing emotional responses generated by this situation. As theories of stress and coping are considered in some detail in Chapter 3, only brief reference is made to these here.

Stress has been described as a phenomenon within which trans-actional and dynamic relationships operate among the person, the situation and the environment (Folkman 1984). When an individual meets with a potentially threatening situation, a primary appraisal is made which enables judgements to be made about whether the situation is non-threatening and therefore needing no further action, or threatening and requiring a coping response. An appraisal–reap-praisal loop follows, within which evaluations are made of the coping resources, and coping strategies are mobilized to counter the threat (Folkman 1984).

Coping strategies consist of the cognitive and behavioural efforts in which individuals engage to control, reduce or tolerate the demands posed by a stressful situation (Folkman 1984). Although the literature is heavily weighted towards identification of relatives' needs and concerns, a few studies have explored relatives' coping responses (Nugent 1988; Woods, Lewis and Ellison 1989; Wilson and Morse 1991; Hull 1992).

Thorne (1985) conducted a small phenomenological study to explore coping strategies of cancer patients' relatives. Relatives' main coping responses included information seeking, mobilizing social support, and intrapsychic defences such as cognitive re-formu-lation and denial (Thorne 1985). In cognitive re-formulation, perceptions of a situation are manipulated in an effort to view the stressful situation in a more positive light. Denial, within the context of terminal illness, usually involves avoiding thinking about or discussing the prognosis, or indeed simply refusing to believe it (Thorne 1985). Thorne's sample was small ($n = 12$) and heteroge-neous in terms of care site, stage of cancer and the relationship of the relative to the patient. Also, the patient and relative were interviewed together which might well have influenced the interviewee's responses. However, these findings have been corroborated elsewhere (Hull 1992). In Hull's study, reported earlier, a range of intrapsychic coping strategies that relatives employ were identified, including cognitive re-formulation, social comparison and denial. 'Time re-formulation' was also reported which allowed goals to be altered to enable relatives to take 'one day at a time'. Social support from family, friends and health-care professionals was also found to represent important coping resources for relatives (Hull 1992). Hull (1992) recommends further research aimed at identifying effective coping strategies for families and using this information to develop nursing interventions to enhance family support.

The research literature on coping has confirmed that intrapsychic defences are commonly used by patients and relatives during the course of a terminal illness.

Denial and hope

Denial is a dynamic coping response that is dependent on contextual factors for its expression over time. It operates as a form of self-deception that protects individuals from threat and exaggerates their perceptions of control and self-efficacy (Russell 1993). During a progressive and fatal illness, the family can be repeatedly thrown into chaos as the illness moves from one stage to another, and denial will also tend to fluctuate as threats wax and wane. Although denial is commonly viewed as a pathological response, it can also operate as a valuable buffer against stress. By blunting the full force of the truth, denial can allow situations to be viewed more positively, thus lowering anxiety, aiding decision-making and 'protecting the self concept against the ultimate threat of disintegration' (Russell 1993). In his literature-based analysis of denial, Russell challenges the view that denial is a maladaptive response. The author claims that, within the context of terminal illness, denial can represent a buffer against hopelessness. He concludes that our psychological health may, in part, be contingent on our ability to view events through an 'illusionary glow' (Russell 1993).

Herth explored the shifting dimensions of hope with dying patients and their caregivers and she defined hope as an 'inner power that facilitates transcendence of the present' (Herth 1990, 1993). Herth's own study employed methodological triangulation using interview data, background data and the Herth Hope Index as data sources; a sample of 25 relatives was recruited from two hospice programmes (Herth 1990, 1993). Findings reveal hope as a significant coping resource, which has transactional properties in that evidence of hope in close family members has a role in maintaining a sense of hopefulness in the dying patient (Herth 1993). Scanlon (1989) similarly describes the dynamic and reciprocal effects that hopefulness or hopelessness in one person within a relationship can have on the others. Herth's (1993) findings about factors that foster hope and those that hinder hope in relatives of dying patients are summarized below.

Hope fostered by

• Sustaining relationships that provide a supportive anchor for the relatives
• Cognitive re-framing that allows threatening perceptions to be transformed into a more positive frame
• Time re-focusing: adjusting to short-term goals by taking one day at a time
• Spiritual beliefs: having belief in a power greater than themselves
• Conserving energy: learning to conserve finite energy reserves to meet the demands posed by the situation.

Hope hindered by

• Isolation: which can be physical, emotional or spiritual
• Concurrent losses: which can lead to emotional overload
• Poorly controlled symptoms: witnessing suffering in a loved one.

According to Herth (1993), nurses can support and sustain hope in relatives, and therefore also in patients, by maintaining a caring presence, offering relatives physical and emotional comfort, ensuring that optimal standards of comfort and care are provided for the patient, and providing regular information for relatives. Herth also urges staff to convey a sense of availability so that a supportive relationship can be formed with the relatives, thus facilitating the preservation of hopefulness in both patient and family (Herth 1993).

    Below further consideration is given to the support needs and coping responses of relatives within the context of communication. As gaining access to information about the patient's condition has consistently been found to be crucial to family coping and support, this area is considered first. Subsequently, an exploration of some of the complex and interrelated communication issues that operate within the context of terminal illness is conducted.

Communication in terminal illness

Information needs

It has been established from the literature that the information needs of relatives of dying patients centre around their need to know that their dying loved one is comfortable, is having adequate symptom control, and is being well cared for and valued as a person (Mayer 1986; Faulkner 1988a; Morris 1988; Farrar 1992; Wilkinson 1992). Hockley, Dunlop and Davies (1988) found that relatives in acute hospital wards experience severe stress when unable to gain access to information, yet despite their reported distress they seemed to accept passively that other pressures on doctors' time preclude them from seeing the family. Difficulties that relatives experience in their communications with hospital doctors, especially around the time of diagnosis and during the terminal period of the patient's illness, have now been widely reported (Maguire and Faulkner 1988; Higginson et al. 1990; Weatherall 1994).

Although the desire for information is particularly high among cancer patients and their families, achieving satisfaction with the provision of information is not entirely straightforward (Steptoe et al. 1991). These authors investigated satisfaction with communication among 77 oncology patients, and found that an individual's psychological coping style represented an important indicator of information needs (Steptoe et al. 1991). The researchers categorized people in terms of their information-seeking behaviour. Some, described as 'information seekers' (or monitors), were found to require copious amounts of information and would report an information deficit even if provided with regular information. In contrast, 'information avoiders' (or blunters) were found to cope by avoiding, or failing to seek out, information. Such people habitually rely on avoidance behaviour or distraction as their usual coping style (Steptoe et al. 1991). Steptoe and colleagues emphasize that these findings must not be taken to imply that information need not be provided, nor that efforts to enhance communication are doomed to fail. On the contrary, they conclude that the case for giving information to cancer patients and their families remains overwhelming. These authors suggest that, if information is given sensitively, people will select the level of detail, and degree of confrontation with the facts, that they require (Steptoe et al. 1991). Fallowfield (1993a) endorses this view, stressing that the provision of information does not preclude the use of denial or other avoidant coping strategies.

Social mores will profoundly affect the communication patterns that surround death and dying. Indeed, in most societies, the dying process tends to be a socially constructed phenomenon supported by unwritten rules that govern the ways in which it should be managed and confronted (Davies 1990; Perakyla 1991). Literature relating to communication in terminal care reveals a complex web of coping strategies employed by all the participants caught up in the situation. A pivotal issue is whether, and by whom, the forthcoming death is acknowledged and accepted, because this will profoundly influence the nature of communications and also raise a number of important ethical issues for health-care professionals (Mitchell 1987; Hunt 1991a; Farrar 1992).

Awareness contexts

It is now more than 30 years since Glaser and Strauss first described the ways in which communication among dying people, their families and those involved in their care are influenced by the level of acknowledgement and acceptance of the forthcoming death (Glaser and Strauss 1965). They used the term 'awareness contexts' to represent a continuum, at one end of which 'closed awareness' is characterized by a failure on the part of all concerned to acknowledge the fatal prognosis. At the opposite end is 'open awareness', where open dialogue occurs among all parties about the impending death. Between these extremes lie the intermediate states of 'suspicion awareness', commonly characterized by the family and caregivers being aware of the prognosis and the patient having unconfirmed suspicions, and 'mutual pretence' where all parties are fully aware of the prognosis but they elect to pretend otherwise (Seale 1991).

The ethics of collusion

Seale revisits awareness contexts and disclosure about death in a study which, although not an exact replication, compares findings with those of an earlier study conducted by Cartwright and others some 20 years previously (Cartwright et al. 1973; Seale 1993). In the later study, relatives, and nursing and medical staff, who had contact with 639 adults whose deaths were registered in England during 1987, were asked their views about communication issues related to care of dying patients (Seale 1993). Findings indicate that, although there has been a move towards more open disclosure of diagnosis, it is still common for relatives to be given the diagnosis first and for the patient not to be told at all. Comparison of different diagnostic groups revealed that cancer patients were most likely to be informed about their prognosis, whereas those with disorders that might impair mental functioning, such as dementia or stroke, were least likely to be told (Seale 1993).

A number of authors have explored the complex and sensitive issues that surround truth telling during terminal illness (Hinton 1981; Youll 1989; Hunt 1991a; Bakhurst 1992; Janes 1992; Shea and Kendrick 1995). A study of awareness of diagnosis in cancer patients who had been referred to symptom control nurses found that 94% of the patients ($n = 50$) were aware that they had cancer, although some openly acknowledged it for the first time with the specialist nurses (Hunt 1991a). In 1990, a Gallup survey revealed that 94% of those polled would want to know the truth about any serious illness that they had (Hodson 1990). Hodson posits that the conspiracy of silence that still surrounds disclosure of prognosis rests on assumptions of doctors and nurses that, if dying patients were to be told the truth, they would simply give up hope. He also claims that staff and relatives often collude to conceal the truth from the patient (Hodson 1990).

The common situation in which relatives know the prognosis but the patient does not has been described as 'the slippery slope to moral quandary' (Shea and Kendrick 1995). Although relatives undoubtedly act from a beneficent perspective when they withhold the truth from the patient, such collusion raises a number of fundamental ethical issues, including those of autonomy, respect, honesty and trust (Shea and Kendrick 1995). Bakhurst (1992) asserts that deception, however benevolent, denies patients due respect and may also deprive them of the opportunity to come to terms with their own mortality and to take their proper leave of family and friends. In a similar vein, Maguire (1985a) claims that collusion can erode the very foundations of a relationship, causing the patient and family to drift apart emotionally, although Hinton (1981), in his study of collusion between spouses, found that couples caught up in such deception were unable to comfort one another, and each partner was left to bear the pain alone. To have to face your own death without the benefit of an honest and trusting relationship could prove an 'alienating and desperate experience' (Shea and Kendrick 1995).

Although the literature underscores the value of open, honest communication during terminal illness, the suggestion that 'open awareness' is universally preferred has been challenged. Some studies reveal that the habitual communication patterns of some families might make open disclosure inappropriate and indeed the secret of some families' success in coping with cancer might well be their decision to avoid open discussion of the prognosis (Thorne 1985; Woods et al. 1989). Weisman also cautions against forcing the truth on those who do not want it, arguing that this can be just as inexcusable as proscribing honest discussions (Weisman 1979). Seale (1991), in a similar vein, describes the enthusiasm that some doctors now have for breaking silence about a fatal prognosis as being like 'a medical interrogation with patients almost being brought to confess their own deaths'. Although imparting a fatal prognosis will never be easy, it should be done gently within a context of support and with the understanding that not everyone wishes to know all (Maguire and Faulkner 1988; Seale 1991; Fallowfield 1993a). Also, in so far as it is possible, efforts should be made to emphasize any positive aspects of the situation (Herth 1990). Shea and Kendrick (1995) argue that care should be taken not to underestimate people's inner resources. Although avoiding deceit remains a basic moral canon, the truth 'need not be breached with a fist of steel, but should rather be embraced by a velvet glove'.

The staff–relative interface

The onus for initiating contact between staff and relatives usually rests with the family, and yet relatives consistently report feeling inhibited about approaching hospital staff whom they perceive as being too busy to spend time with them. The need for staff to convey a sense of availability to the dying patient's family has now been widely reported (Hackett and Weisman 1985; Hull 1989a; Lugton 1989a).

Dunlop and Hockley (1990) found that around 50% of relatives of dying patients in hospital did not see a doctor at all during their loved one's final admission. Reasons suggested for these low levels of contact include relatives' hesitancy about approaching staff, the fact that medical staff are rarely around the wards during visiting times and that nurses are perceived as being either too busy or lacking the authority to answer their questions (Dunlop and Hockley 1990). As it is also possible that the low levels of staff–relative contact may, in part, be the result of avoidance behaviour in staff, this area is considered below.

Social forces appear to pressurize health professionals into controlling, denying and hiding from death (Farrar 1992). Wilkinson (1991) explored communication patterns of registered nurses in both specialist and non-specialist hospitals by analysing audio-taped interviews of the nurses undertaking case histories with cancer patients who were (1) newly diagnosed, (2) admitted with recurrence or (3) receiving palliative care. Nurses in both settings were frequently found to exhibit conversation-blocking techniques in response to the patients' efforts to discuss their concerns. Overall, facilitative communication was found to be poor and this was most notable with patients experiencing recurrence of their disease. Of the nurses 70% admitted taking avoiding action when communicating with dying patients and their families (Wilkinson 1991).

There is no doubt that to be regularly confronted with death and faced with the grief of others can be painful and emotionally demanding. It is therefore not surprising that nurses will seek ways of protecting themselves; indeed the distancing and avoidance behaviour that many nurses employ when caring for patients with a poor prognosis are now well documented (Maguire 1988; Doyle 1991; Kelsey 1992; Weatherall 1994).

The ward climate

Field (1984) confirms that the ward environment will exert an influence on how staff respond to dying patients and their families. Nurses in wards in which death is an infrequent and unpredictable event report higher levels of stress than nurses in wards where death is a more common occurrence. In addition, staff also find it stressful when a young person dies, especially in the case of a child (Field

1984). Aspects of ward organization and the leadership style of the charge nurse have also been found to influence communication patterns among nurses, patients and relatives during terminal illness (Field 1984; Northouse and Northouse 1987; Seale 1991; Steptoe et al. 1991; Wilkinson 1991). In particular, Wilkinson (1991) reported that the climate created by the ward sister significantly influenced the nature and style of communication in hospital especially during terminal illness.

Field (1984) interviewed nurses in an acute medical ward in order to explore aspects of hospital care during terminal illness. The ward was run on team nursing lines with widely delegated authority and autonomy. A policy of open disclosure operated and nurses were free to answer patients' and relatives' questions about diagnosis and prognosis (Field 1984). All but two participants stated a preference for open disclosure. The qualified nurses all reported having developed strategies for telling patients the truth, although the ward sister was sometimes called upon to help negotiate the delicate path to open awareness. Students' and auxiliaries' communication strategies differed and tended to rely on conversation control and avoidance tactics (Field 1984). This finding is particularly significant in the light of reports that care of dying patients in hospitals is largely carried out by untrained staff (Knight 1981; Melia 1982). Nurses in Field's (1984) study all reported having become emotionally involved, to the point of grieving when a patient died, and such involvement usually meant that they also became involved with the family. The level of anxiety that involvement with the family generated was higher in unqualified staff.

Field, with a co-researcher (Knight), also investigated terminal care in an acute surgical ward (Knight 1981). The surgical ward, in contrast to the medical ward reported above, was run on formal hierarchical lines, had a rapid turnover of patients and operated a 'strictly routinized' approach to care. A 'decision rule' existed to withhold information from patients, and staff, relatives and other patients colluded in this deception. Most of the direct care was given by students and auxiliaries, and distancing and avoidance strategies were commonly observed (Field 1984). Field posits that staff exposed to such negative experiences can experience a loss of idealism, which can lead them to develop an attitude of detached concern. Conversely, Field argues that when the ward leadership style fosters a commitment to caring for the whole person, the job satisfaction and rewards that flow from this can work to the benefit of patients, relatives and staff.

Comparing these findings is, however, problematic because the researchers' relationship with staff and patients differed within each setting. In the medical ward, interviews with nursing staff represented the main reported data source, whereas on the surgical ward covert participant observation methods were employed. One of the investigators (Knight) worked as a nursing auxiliary during data gathering without the knowledge of most of the staff (Knight 1981). The samples were also small and heterogeneous, in that they comprised both qualified nurses and unqualified staff. Despite these possible limitations, and although Field and Knight's findings are now more than 10 years old, the communication and interprofessional issues that they raise remain salient.

The professional carer's perspective

Interprofessional relationships

The complex relationships that operate between the medical and nursing professions have received wide comment in the literature (Altschul 1983; Crowley and Wollner 1987; Fraser 1988; Kennedy and Garvin 1988; Iles and Auluck 1990). Synthesis of this literature reveals that, where collaborative and collegial relationships exist, effective communication and trust are enhanced, leading to a reduction in interprofessional tension. Collaborative initiatives have been found to benefit patients by virtue of the improved working atmosphere and better coordinated care that result (Crowley and Wollner 1987). Interprofessional collaboration is facilitated in environments that are receptive to change and where the motivation to improve interprofessional communication is high (Crowley and Wollner 1987). This is confirmed by Iles and Auluck (1990), who draw on their experience in industry and with a community drugs team to explore the development of interdisciplinary teamwork in health care. The authors conclude that effective interprofessional collaboration relies on mutual trust and respect, effective channels of communication, and the motivation and commitment to cooperate (Iles and Auluck 1990).

Field (1984), reporting on aspects of interprofessional communication in hospital, asserts that hospital doctors control the information that nurses can give to patients and relatives, and indeed nurses may actually be forbidden to reveal that a patient is dying. Although Field acknowledges that communications are often less hierarchical and formal than this, he insists that in the final instance decision-making in hospital still rests firmly with the doctor. This finding is corroborated by Seale who compared the findings from two studies conducted some 20 years apart (Cartwright et al. 1973; Seale 1993). Although nurses in the later study perceived that they had greater freedom to answer questions, a significant number of both doctors and nurses still judged that it would be inappropriate for nurses to divulge information about diagnosis, prognosis or treatment (Seale 1993).

Such findings raise questions about the position that nurses hold within the health-care team, and in particular raise issues relating to the extent to which nurses can claim to be autonomous and able to act as advocates for their patients and their families. Although the UKCC Code of Professional Conduct requires all registered nurses to 'act always in such a way as to promote and safeguard the well-being and interests of patients and clients' (UK Central Council 1992), Sutor (1993) argues that nurses, constrained by the patriarchal nature of the medical profession, have yet to realize the professional autonomy that this degree of advocacy requires.

Although the employment pattern is changing, nursing has historically recruited predominantly young women who are motivated to nurture and care (Maslin-Prothero 1992; Waterson 1992). Field (1984) suggests that it is this feminine basis of nursing that contributes significantly to the subordinate position that nurses hold within the hospital hierarchy. Also, commenting on the paternalistic nature of the relationships between doctors and their patients and between the medical and nursing professions, Holden (1991) describes how nurses can become caught up in collusion and deception, especially during a patient's terminal illness. She expresses this view as follows:

> If doctors ceased the practice of making unrealistic promises to patients then they would no longer need to abandon their patients to pre-mortem loneliness and nurses would henceforth be able to enjoy greater medical support when caring for the dying patient.
>
> (Holden 1991, p. 403)

The professional constraints that are imposed on their communications with the dying patient and family have been found to generate stress in nurses (Holden 1991).

Nurses' stress

Psychiatric morbidity associated with stress in nursing is reported by a number of authors (Hingley and Harris 1986a; Maguire 1988; Nash 1989; Hiscox 1991; Nganasurian 1992). In particular, it has been reported that nurses top the list for psychiatric outpatient referrals and, when compared with other professional groups, nurses smoke more, drink more, have a high rate of absenteeism and an alarmingly high suicide rate (Hingley and Harris 1986a; Cole 1992).

Alexander (1990) studied stress in palliative care nurses working in two specialist units in Scotland. The sample comprised 61 full- and part-time nurses from both day and night duty. None of these hospice nurses had undertaken any form of specialist training. Stress associated with dealing with relatives was reported by 64% of the nurses, and most believed that they had received inadequate preparation for this aspect of their role (Alexander 1990). Although admitting the limitations imposed by the sample size and lack of a comparison group, Alexander suggests the need for research and education aimed at developing: (1) favourable attitudes to terminal care in nurses, (2) realistic expectations in nurses to reduce feelings of failure and helplessness and (3) supportive professional working relationships within the palliative care setting.

Benoliel and colleagues (1990) used a Nurse Stress Checklist (NSC) to explore the nature of stress in nursing. Based on a transactional model of stress, this instrument measures stress as a multidimensional construct (Lazarus and Folkman 1984). The sample of 104 staff was drawn from a variety of clinical settings within an American urban community.

Factor analysis revealed the main components of the nurses' stress related to:

(1) personal reactions to stress, including emotional, cognitive and physical responses
(2) role conflicts experienced within their personal and professional life
(3) work related concerns which included:
  • interprofessional relationships

- work environment which included resources, staffing and facilities
- concerns about their own abilities to keep up with work demands.

(Benoliel et al. 1990, p. 226)

The multifaceted character of clinical stress, which Benoliel's findings demonstrate, confirms that stress associated with providing terminal care is closely linked to concurrent stresses such as home or family conflicts, work-related conflicts, and excessive and conflicting role demands (Benoliel et al. 1990). The female nurse, especially with dependent children, has been found to be particularly vulnerable to stress and conflict as a result of the dual demands of home and work (Hingley and Harris 1986a; Nganasurian 1992). Stress and burnout are now commonly experienced by nurses, especially those who work in acute care settings (Oberle and Davies 1992).

The roots of burnout

The dominance of the medical model and of task-oriented approaches to nursing care, which have held sway for so long, create philosophical difficulties for nurses who wish to practise within a humanistic framework but who work in high-technology areas (Oberle and Davies 1993). Central to the humanistic approach is the notion that each person is a unitary being who cannot be reduced to component parts and whose unique personhood must be respected. Caring theories that reflect this philosophy have been explicated by a growing body of nursing scholars (Benner and Wrubel 1989; Watson 1990; Oberle and Davies 1992; Saunders and Valente 1994; Parse 1995).

Oberle and Davies (1993) used a grounded theory approach and the experiences of expert nurses in palliative care to explore the roots of disillusionment and burnout in nursing. The investigators found that, when a nurse's personal belief system is rooted in a humanistic caring ethic but the working environment is not conducive to that type of care, the nurse's personal values are compromised and cognitive dissonance results. Dissonance creates such discomfort that individuals will go to considerable lengths to reduce it (Oberle and Davies 1993). Within the terminal care context, such measures might include the nurse engaging in distancing and avoidance behaviour with the patient and family. Oberle and Davies (1993) suggest that, when nurses are frustrated in their attempts to deliver care that is congruent with their personal values, they can be deprived of the primary source of satisfaction and energy that provides them with the strength to continue, despite the high emotional cost of caring. In such circumstances nurses can become emotionally exhausted, disillusioned and 'burned out'. Benner and Wrubel (1988) concur with this contention, arguing that it is a 'peculiarly modern mistake' to suggest that caring is the cause of burnout and that the cure is to protect oneself from caring by avoidance behaviour. These authors assert that in reality burnout comes through a loss of caring capacity and indeed the return of caring is needed for recovery from burnout.

Benner and Wrubel also argue that coping (or indeed *not* coping) with care-giving must be considered within the full context of nursing in society. Nurses in acute care daily confront life-threatening situations and complicated treatment regimens that leave little margin for error. Stress in nursing can arise from the array of demands imposed on nurses as they strive to keep abreast of the knowledge explosion, while working in complex organizations in which they often lack professional recognition or reward and often in the face of chronic staff shortages. Although disengagement may blunt the emotional pain that such cumulative stresses engender, recovery will require rest, respite, and the reintegration of human concern and involvement (Benner and Wrubel 1988).

Whether humanistic approaches to care are the cause of, or indeed the solution to, stress and burnout in palliative care is open to debate. It has been argued that nurses who regularly care for dying patients, using approaches such as primary nursing to reduce the emotional distance between nurse and patient, can experience bereavement overload, leading to stress and burnout (Firth et al. 1987; Fisher 1988; Saunders and Valente 1994). Within the dynamic context of the relationships that operate among nurses and patients and families, it is possible that there are optimum levels of involvement that facilitate compassionate care while preserving the emotional safety of the professional carer (Cherniss 1980; Ceslowitz 1989).

Whether work-related stress in palliative nursing will lead to burnout, a career change or the implementation of constructive coping activity will depend, in part, on the nurse's ability to face her or his own mortality and to accept her or his emotional responses to death (Saunders and Valente 1994). These authors suggest that nurses need to develop 'emotional muscle' to enable them to cope effectively with the demands imposed by this type of care.

In a similar vein, Harper and Fulton (1977) offer a model to describe the emotional adaptation processes that nurses go through when they are regularly exposed to death and grief. Harper's model, explicated by Fisher (1988), describes five stages of emotional growth. These stages (summarized below) do not necessarily occur sequentially or within any prescribed timescale (Fisher 1988).

Harper's schematic growth and development scale

- Intellectualization: the focus is on factual and procedural matters. Brisk activity and superficial communications are usual
- Emotional trauma/survival: this involves the discomfort of facing own mortality. Guilt and frustration are common at this stage
- Depression, pain and mourning: at this crucial stage the nurse must decide to 'go or grow' (or use distancing/avoidance tactics)
- Emotional arrival: the nurse, although still sad when a patient dies, can accommodate the grief and is no longer preoccupied with own health or death
- Deep compassion and self-actualization: the nurse can now relate openly compassionately to the dying patient and family and is able to offer humane, professional care.

(Harper and Fulton 1977)

Professional depression or 'burnout' is essentially a response to unrelenting stress experienced within a context of inadequate resources, and inadequate staff preparation and support (Cole 1992).

Stress management in nursing

Given the wide range of personal, interpersonal and organizational factors that underpin occupational stress in nursing, it is likely that stress management will require a multi-dimensional approach (Hingley and Harris 1986a). Such an approach to stress management might include personal coping strategies, such as social support from family, peers and colleagues, coping measures such as smoking or drinking alcohol, self-nurturing activities such as relaxation and leisure pursuits, and active problem management approaches.

Stress management may also require access to resources such as counselling, support groups, training initiatives and management support. Responsibility for managing occupational stress and maintaining the health of staff should, therefore, reflect the transactional relationship between the individual and the organization (Hiscox 1991).

The role of education

Doyle (1991) reviewed the provision of palliative education in the UK and describes the expanding role of the hospice movement as an educational catalyst and enabler. He argues for the benefits of inter-disciplinary educational effort at all stages of training and practice. Doyle suggests that attendance at courses is limited, not by the number of enthusiastic would-be students, but by economic and other resource constraints which operate within the current climate in the NHS.

Lyons (1988) surveyed 39 clinical nurses and 26 nurse teachers about their education needs in relation to care of the dying. She found that 56% of clinical nursing staff experienced stress when communicating with dying patients and their relatives, and 90% expressed a need for additional teaching in this area. Although the small sample size limits the generalizability of these findings, the literature offers ample corroboration of nurses' unmet needs for access to additional training, particularly in the areas of communication and counselling (Lugton 1987; Hyde 1988; Hockley 1989; Kelsey 1992). Faulkner (1988a) cogently argues that, if nurses are taught interactional skills with patients, relatives and colleagues, then stress, ill-health and burnout in staff can be significantly reduced.

The literature is rich in comment about the potential that educational interventions hold for reducing the anxiety that nurses experience when providing care for dying patients and their families (Doyle 1987; Degner and Gow 1988a; Hinds 1989; Kristjanson and Scanlan 1989; Corner and Wilson-Barnett 1992; Fallowfield 1993a; Farrell 1993). However, Degner and Gow (1988a) also underline the paucity of convincing evaluation research to support claims made for specific educational approaches (Degner and Gow 1988a). The authors conducted a quasi-experimental study with a sample of 306 undergraduate nurses in the USA, to evaluate the effects that different educational approaches had on nurse anxiety when caring for dying patients (Degner and Gow 1988a). When compared with the control group at one year after graduation, it was found that the experimental group, who had been exposed to an integrated theory/practice model and had used experiential learning methods, reported less anxiety and more 'approach behaviours' when caring for dying patients (Degner and Gow 1988a).

These findings are supported in a UK study that used a combined questionnaire and interview approach to identify attitudes to cancer and the educational needs of 127 newly registered nurses (Corner and Wilson-Barnett 1992). Findings revealed that nurses hold deep concerns about caring for patients with cancer and consider themselves to be ill-prepared for this aspect of their role. Knowledge about cancer was also found to be poor. The study compared the impact of different educational strategies in three groups of nurses: group 1 attended a formal seminar teaching programme; group 2 were exposed to experiential workshops; and group 3 formed the non-intervention control group. The most obvious change related to nurses' increased confidence in communication and psychological care for dying patients. This was reported by 75.6% of the experiential workshop group, 44% of the seminar group and 12.5% of the control group (Corner and Wilson-Barnett 1992). These findings underscore the encouraging potential that experiential learning initiatives offer to nurse education in this area. It must, however, be acknowledged that other studies that have sought to establish sustained benefits of education on nurses' anxiety and communication during terminal illness behaviour have produced equivocal findings (Chodil and Dulaney 1984; Wilkinson 1991).

Counselling and support

While acknowledging the need for individual responsibility, self-regulation and stress management, researchers working in the field consistently argue for organizational support for staff which should include effective and receptive management and adequate provision of staff and resources (Hingley 1984; Hingley and Harris 1986a, b).

Although the literature relating to counselling in health care is weighted heavily towards the patients' and clients' perspective, staff needs for counselling receive only scant attention (Faulkner, Webb and Maguire 1991; Fallowfield 1993a; Farrell 1993; Moynihan 1993). A number of authors, commenting on the supportive benefits of mentorship and preceptorship for students and newly qualified staff nurses, suggest that *all* staff might benefit from professional mentorship, from someone who would listen openly, challenge constructively and guide supportively (Hingley and Harris 1986a; Armitage and Burnard 1991; Winters 1992).

Hingley and Harris (1986a) advocate the development of peer support initiatives that offer opportunities for staff collectively to engage in problem-solving and collaboration. They suggest that 'quality circles', originally formulated to deal with specific work-related problems, offer an avenue for interprofessional collaboration and reciprocal support, and they also advocate the need to incorporate stress awareness and stress-reduction training into pre- and post-registration nursing education (Hingley and Harris 1986a). The authors finally, and emphatically, argue for the provision of independent support in the form of comprehensive counselling services for nurses.

The stigma of stress

The ambivalence that exists towards occupational stress in nursing leads to the tendency either to deny it or to attribute it to individual weakness. This suggests that nurses need to change their attitudes towards themselves and to each other (Hingley and Harris 1986a, b). Bacon (1993) delivers a simple but crucial message when he observes 'you can't care if you don't feel'. The author describes a hospital-based support group for staff who regularly care for dying patients, and he strongly argues that access to such a facility might just help to sustain staff through periods of difficulty that might otherwise 'force the personal and professional tragedy of a health worker brought to the knees'.

Summary and conclusions

The literature has revealed that increasing numbers of families are being challenged by a diagnosis of cancer within their immediate family circle. Despite improved survival rates, cancer remains one of the main causes of death in the UK. This has implications for the provision of care for people with advanced disease. Despite burgeoning developments in specialist care provision, the literature confirms that, although patients with advanced cancer commonly receive care in more than one setting, most still die in hospital wards.

Literature that describes relatives' needs, concerns and experiences of care in different settings is weighted heavily towards the North American context. The main focus of the literature is on the family caregiver in a home-care context. Studies overwhelmingly reveal that care-giving relatives experience significant stress and have unmet needs for support. A few, small, mainly descriptive, studies that focus on the UK hospice situation were reported, which reveal a higher level of satisfaction with care and communication.

Hospice care in the USA and Canada differs from UK provision, in that it mainly relates to outpatient or day-care facilities supported by specialist doctors and nurses. Studies in these settings, mainly using phenomenological and ethnomethodological approaches with small samples, have provided revealing insights into the experiences, concerns and needs of families with a terminally ill member. Studies that explored the experiences of relatives of terminally ill patients in hospital, particularly within the UK context, are sparsely represented and comprise mainly small-scale descriptive studies, which reveal that access to staff and information represent significant concerns for relatives in hospital.

Literature that focused on the issues surrounding communication during terminal illness provided useful analysis of such issues as information needs, disclosure of prognosis, collusion, denial and hope. A number of major UK reports were uncovered which contribute significantly to the body of knowledge in these important areas (Higginson et al. 1990; Seale 1991; Steptoe et al. 1991; Wilkinson 1991; Herth 1993).

The transactional nature of stress and coping, and of communication, was clearly highlighted in the literature. The interlinked and overarching themes of stress and communication permeated the entire body of the literature. Despite this persuasive evidence of stress as a major issue in this field of study, only a few examples emerged in which stress and coping were used as a theoretical framework to underpin the research work. One UK study that did employ a stress and coping framework focused on the cancer nurses' perspective and did not specifically focus on the issue of relatives' needs (E Hanson 1994).

A considerable volume of research was uncovered which explores and describes relatives' needs and concerns, but little evidence was found of intervention work designed to address these needs and concerns. One exception was a small-scale American study, conducted some 17 years ago, which used another researcher's findings (Hampe 1975) to design and evaluate an intervention to improve support for the families of dying patients in a coronary care unit (Dracup and Breu 1978).

Literature that reports the nurses' perspective focuses almost entirely on the causes and effects of stress and burnout, and nurses' needs for resources, support and education (Hingley 1984; Baglioni, Cooper and Hingley 1990; Seale 1992). A large body of literature was uncovered that describes the difficulties that nurses experience in their communications with dying patients and their families, and the coping responses that they employ. A recent UK study, which analysed nurses' avoidance behaviour in communications with cancer patients, makes a significant contribution to knowledge in this area (Wilkinson 1991). However, communication with relatives did not feature in this research work.

Only one example has been found of a study that attempts to explore the dual perspectives of the dying patient's relatives and the nurses who provide care (Wros 1993). This exploratory phenomenological study was conducted within a critical care setting in the USA and the study design did not incorporate an intervention. No evidence has been found in either the UK or the US literature of any study that seeks to elicit the dual perspectives of nurses and relatives of families of dying patients in general hospital wards.

An intervention study that seeks the perspectives of both nurses and relatives, and that uses emerging data to design, implement and evaluate an intervention aimed at improving family care and support during terminal illness would therefore represent an original contribution to the body of nursing knowledge in this field.

Chapter 3
The theoretical
framework

The literature has revealed that terminal illness imposes considerable stress on both families and professionals (Birch 1979; Faulkner and Maguire 1988; Ceslowitz 1989; McWhan 1991; Wilkinson 1992). It was therefore considered that a deeper understanding of stress and coping theories would enable the full extent of the stress experience and individual ways of dealing with the stress to be taken into account. It was also judged that conducting the study within a stress and coping framework might facilitate a coherent approach to data gathering and to the comparative evaluation of interview data before and after intervention.

Theories of stress are commonly described in relation to their associated models. Stress may therefore be described in terms of external stimuli that impinge upon an individual (stimulus-based model), an individual's physical and psychological reactions to a stressor (response-based model) or in relation to the dynamic interplay that operates among the individual, the situation and the environment (transactional model). Each of these models is described below.

Models of stress and coping

Stimulus-based models

Proponents of stimulus-based models of stress assume that external stressors are brought to bear on individuals, causing them to experience strain (Bailley and Clark 1989). The most commonly cited stimulus-based model is the 'strain–stress' model. Its roots are in engineering theory and, in particular, Hooke's law of elasticity, which describes how deformations occur in metals that are exposed to an excessive load or force (*International Dictionary in Physics* 1961). Bailley and Clark (1989) argue that such an analogy does not offer a particularly fruitful line of enquiry when seeking to understand the human stress experience. Implicit in the stress–strain model is the expectation that stress will increase in proportion to the level of the external stimulus that is applied, and it is here that the analogy with human stress breaks down, because one of the most disagreeable human experiences is the complete absence of stimuli.

Stressful stimuli might include hunger, extremes of temperature, excessive work load or perhaps, for patients and relatives, exposure to the hospital environment. Holmes and Rahe (1967) developed a rating scale that measures the relative impact of a range of stressful stimuli associated with events in life such as marriage, moving house, serious illness or bereavement (Holmes and Rahe 1967). Attempting to quantify stress in this way is, however, problematic because, although stress might indeed originate from a particularly intense stimulus, it may also be generated by cumulative pressures arising from multiple stressful stimuli (Clarke 1984). The stress–strain model is also based on the assumption that stimuli will uniformly produce strain in all people (Bailley and Clarke 1989). Furthermore, in the metal analogy offered in the stress–strain model, resistance (of the metal) to the applied force is passive, which equates poorly with the dynamic, diverse, coping behaviours that humans engage in when responding to stressful stimuli (Lazarus and Folkman 1984).

In summary, stimulus-based theories of stress have been widely used to support legislation governing a range of environmental stressors, such as noise and air pollution, and as such they have contributed to improved living and working conditions (Leefarr and Cutler 1994). It would, however, be an oversimplification to describe stress purely in terms of noxious stimuli, when it is evident that individuals and their unique circumstances will significantly determine the extent to which given stimuli generate strain (Clarke 1984). Furthermore, it is not possible accurately to identify stimuli that will uniformly cause strain in *all* individuals or, indeed, that will cause strain in the *same* individual on different occasions (Bailley and Clarke 1989). Finally, the simple cause–effect relationship that underpins the stimulus-based model of stress fails to acknowledge the capacity of human beings to take action to cope with their situation, and it therefore offers little promise as a framework for exploring the complexities of the experiences of relatives of dying patients and of the nurses who provide care.

Response-based model

In the response-based model, the main focus of interest is not the stimulus but rather the individuals' responses to given stressors (Bailley and Clarke 1989). It should be noted that stimulus-based and response-based models apply the term 'stress' differently. In the former, stress refers to the noxious stimuli to which the individual is subjected (stress = cause) whereas, in the latter, the source of the stress is termed the 'stressor" and the individual's experience or response is described as stress (stress = effect) (Clarke 1984).

Hans Selye, an eminent endocrinologist, developed a model that focuses mainly on physiological responses to stressors (Selye 1974). Selye characterizes the stress response in terms of a 'general adaptation syndrome' (GAS) which he describes as having three phases, namely alarm, resistance and exhaustion. The *alarm phase* is represented by a cognitive awareness of threat. This generates feelings of alarm accompanied by increased secretion of stress hormones and activity of the autonomic nervous system. This, in turn, causes wide-ranging physiological responses, including superficial vasoconstriction that results in pallor and an increase in blood pressure, heart rate and respiratory rate. These physiological changes, designed to equip the individual to respond to the stress, disrupt the equilibrium of the internal environment. During the *resistance phase*, efforts to restore homoeostasis are initiated. Resistance essentially represents 'physiological coping'. If, however, the stressed state is sustained over a prolonged period of time, the capacity for physiological resistance may be exceeded and the *exhaustion* phase is reached. Organ damage and symptoms of ill-health can occur which, in extreme situations, might even lead to death (Clarke 1984; Dewe 1987; Bailley and Clarke 1989; Nixon 1993; Leefarr and Cutler 1994).

Selye's work was highly influential in early stress research and is still cited in the literature on stress-related illness (Nixon 1993). Selye's model has, however, been criticized for its strong biomedical

orientation and for its failure to address adequately the psychological, social and environmental context within which stress occurs (Folkman and Lazarus 1980; Folkman 1984; Lazarus and Folkman 1984;
Monet and Lazarus 1985). Although some understanding of the
physiological consequences of stress might prove useful when exploring aspects of the relatives' general health and well-being, this somewhat reductionist model fails to recognize the wider psychosocial
components of a stress experience. It would not, therefore, offer an
adequate framework for exploring the relatives' and nurses' experiences or for identifying their coping and support needs. Current
views of stress build on Selye's model, but also take account of the
ability of individuals to interact with their physical and social environment, thereby acknowledging the transactional and dynamic
nature of stress and coping (Clarke 1984).

The transactional model

Lazarus's transactional model of stress and coping adopts a holistic
view, recognizing stress as a unique experience within which personal,
situational and environmental factors will operate in a dynamic and
reflexive manner. This model rests on a cognitive–phenomenological
transactional theory of stress and coping developed by Lazarus and
others (Folkman and Lazarus 1980; Wrubel et al. 1981; Lazarus and
Folkman 1984). Central to the transactional model is the notion of
cognitive appraisal. This represents a subjective, and ongoing, process
through which a situation or event is evaluated with respect to the
degree of threat or harm that it poses and the range of the options that
are available to counter the threat (Folkman and Lazarus 1980;
Lazarus and Folkman 1984). Once primary appraisal of a situation or
event has deemed it to be stressful, secondary appraisal, which involves
an evaluation of available coping options and resources, immediately
follows. In the light of secondary appraisal, perceptions of threat may
be modified and emotional response may change (Bailley and Clarke
1989).

The way in which each person appraises stressful situations will
be influenced by his or her own values, beliefs and attitudes, usual
coping style, the context within which the stress is experienced, and
the availability of coping resources and support (Wrubel et al. 1981;
McHaffie 1992).

Coping styles and strategies

Coping represents not one response but a complex ongoing struggle involving a constellation of processes. The main aims of coping are to take steps (1) to manage the stressful situations (problem-focused coping) and (2) to regulate feelings of distress that arise from such situations (emotion-focused coping) (Folkman and Lazarus 1980).

Problem-focused coping

This usually involves positive action and is used in situations where there is some potential to eliminate, modify or control the source of the stress. This coping mode has also been referred to as 'direct coping' (Clarke 1984) or 'direct action' (Lazarus 1976). Measures taken to counter the threat will be influenced by individuals' personal appraisal of the nature and degree of the threat, by aspects of the situation and environment within which the stress is occurring, and by the range of coping options and resources that are available (Lazarus 1985). The coping response that is generated will therefore be based on the individual's subjective appraisal of the threat and the potential this has for amelioration. In situations deemed not amenable to change, 'purposeful inaction' (Wrubel et al. 1981) or inhibition of action (Lazarus 1985) might also represent a wholly rational response. Indeed, when further problem-solving efforts are deemed to be pointless, emotion-focused (palliative) approaches might offer the only appropriate coping response (Wrubel et al. 1981).

Emotion-focused coping

The aim in emotion-focused coping is to alter the individual's perceptions of a situation in order to reduce the degree of threat that it presents, and to regulate the distressing emotions that it generates. Clarke (1984) would call this 'indirect' or 'palliative' coping, whereas Lazarus (1976) refers to this as 'cognitive coping'. The term 'cognitive coping' encompasses a range of psychological strategies which include denial and avoidance. Psychological defence mechanisms are used liberally by most well-functioning people in the management of their everyday life stresses. Such mechanisms operate in a protective fashion to allow individuals to control the emotional impact of stressful situations (Wrubel et al. 1981).

The literature has revealed that, when relatives are faced with the imminent loss of their loved one, strategies such as denial may represent their only coping option (Russell 1993; Shea and Kendrick 1995). Similarly, staff who are unable to offer any further hope of recovery may resort to avoidance behaviour to protect themselves from the discomfort that such situations generate (Maguire 1985a; Hiscox 1991).

Lazarus's transactional–phenomenological model of stress formed the framework for a study which explored the coping responses employed by a sample of 100 middle-aged men and women in the management of stressful events in their daily lives (Folkman and Lazarus 1980). Findings indicate that emotion-focused and problem-focused measures were employed in combination in 98% of reported stressful episodes. This corroborates findings of Pearlin and Schooler (1978), who report that emotion- and problem-focused coping responses tend to be used synchronously.

In Folkman's study, the context within which stress occurred and the way that the situation was appraised emerged as the most potent determining factors (Folkman and Lazarus 1980). Problem-focused responses were used more in work-related contexts and in situations appraised as having some scope for amelioration. Sex differences were evident, with men reporting more problem-focused and information-seeking responses in the management of work-related stress. However, contrary to cultural stereotypes, no sex differences emerged in the use of emotion-focused coping responses (Folkman and Lazarus 1980). These findings are at variance with those of Pearlin and Schooler (1978), who found that effective coping was unevenly distributed, with men, and educated and affluent people making greater use of efficacious (problem-focused) strategies.

Pearlin and Schooler's (1978) large multi-phase American investigation ($n = 2300$) into coping strategies employed in different social roles revealed that coping has three main purposes. Coping efforts tend to be directed at (1) modifying the stressful situation, (2) modifying the individual's perception of the situation and (3) managing the emotional response to the stress. The protective function of coping was found to work best in close interpersonal roles such as child rearing and marriage, and was least effective in managing occupational stress (Pearlin and Schooler 1978). This study has been criticized for its focus on unresolved life strains to the exclusion of successfully

managed stresses, and for seeking *general* rather than specific examples of stressful encounters and coping responses (Folkman and
Lazarus 1980).

Influences on coping

Within every stressful encounter, dynamic and reciprocal factors will
operate among the person, the situation and the environment. Coping
efforts will occur within this transactional context and will be influenced by factors within the situation, the environment and the person.

Factors within the situation

In unique or strange situations, individuals can lack the knowledge
needed to guide them towards appropriate coping skills. In the situation of impending loss within the strange and potentially intimidating hospital environment, relatives of dying patients may experience
feelings of helplessness and loss of control, thus rendering them
vulnerable to stress and breakdown (Wrubel et al. 1981). Furthermore, situations that are unremitting in character have also been
found to undermine coping resources and to lead to exhaustion.
Protracted terminal illness is precisely the sort of situation that,
because of its unrelenting nature, can cause increasing levels of stress
in families (Gregory and English 1994).

Serious illness and bereavement are all pervading in their character and as such they present a major challenge to the individual's
coping capacity (Hackett and Weisman 1985; McGhee 1994).
Finally, when the nature and severity of a situation are ambiguous
and unpredictable, this is generally perceived as highly stressful
(Wrubel et al. 1981; Benner and Wrubel 1989).

Factors within the environment

The literature confirms that, in the hospital setting, where events
might be experienced by patients and relatives as alien and unpredictable, stress can be moderated and coping resources supported by
the provision of information (Kristjanson 1986; Morris 1988;
Lugton 1989a). Information-seeking behaviour during terminal
illness has been widely studied (Janis 1983; Seale 1991; Steptoe et al.
1991). Although there is substantial evidence to indicate that,

although for most people information provides a sense of personal efficacy and control, for others it might threaten intrapsychic defences such as denial and avoidance (Steptoe et al. 1991). There is also evidence that individuals will, to some extent, exercise choice in the extent to which they seek, use or reject, information as a coping resource (Janis 1983).

A number of theorists have described information-seeking behaviour using descriptive terms such as 'vigilants' and 'deniers' (Monet and Lazarus 1985), 'monitors' and 'blunters' (Steptoe et al. 1991), and 'hyper-vigilants', 'vigilants' and 'defensive avoiders' (Janis 1983). Despite the apparent disparity in information needs that such terms convey, the authors emphasize that the case for giving information remains overwhelming. Indeed, Janis (1983) asserts that, if communications are sensitively handled, people will be able to select the level and detail of information that they feel able to accommodate. Fallowfield (1993a) concurs with this argument that the provision of information does not prevent or preclude the use of denial and other avoidance strategies.

Information-seeking behaviour is intricately linked with the stress–appraisal loop, which is a central feature of the transactional model of stress and coping (Folkman 1984). As new information is obtained, it is fed into the system enabling reappraisals to be made in the light of changing options and resources. This has implications for nursing practice because it suggests that, by using sensitive communication techniques, it should be possible to support the coping efforts of patients and relatives (Stedeford 1981; Maguire 1985). Supportive social relations, including family, friends and co-workers, also profoundly influence an individual's coping effectiveness (Pearlin and Schooler 1978; Wrubel et al. 1981). This has particular relevance within hospital practice where patients, especially when gravely ill, can feel cut off from their family who usually represent their primary source of support (Hackett and Weisman 1985). By ensuring that relatives are made welcome and comfortable in the ward, nurses may also be enhancing the dying patient's comfort and well-being.

Factors within the person

The significance that a situation or event holds for each person will be determined largely by the personal values, beliefs and commitments that integrate the individual into his or her social world (Bailley and Clarke 1989; McHaffie 1992). This complex range of influences, described as the individual's 'psychological constellation of beliefs', is constantly revised, differentiated and developed in the light of new demands (Bailley and Clarke 1989). Unpredictable or catastrophic events, such as the impending death of a loved one, can cause such devastation and loss of control that a whole new constellation of beliefs may need to be constructed (Bailley and Clarke 1989). The literature offers convincing evidence that many, though not all, people exposed to severe sustained stress such as that generated by fatal illness in a loved one exhibit physical and psychiatric ill-health (Weisman 1979; Nixon 1993; Larsson et al. 1994; McGhee 1994).

In an effort to understand the complex range of factors that help people cope with potentially devastating circumstances, Antonovsky (1987) studied both survivors of the holocaust and also impoverished black Americans. He noted that some people, despite being subjected to significant stress, appeared to suffer no lasting physical or psychological damage. This led him to question 'whence the strength?' (Strumpfer 1990) and stimulated him further to study the phenomenon of 'salutogenesis', which refers to the apparent resistance to developing stress-induced pathology that some individuals exhibit. Within the context of stress and coping, the term 'salutogenesis' is contrasted with 'pathogenesis', where physiological or psychological harm results from exposure to stress (Strumpfer 1990). Antonovsky posited that people who seemed to have 'survived' stress apparently unscathed had called upon a whole range of physiological, economic, cognitive, emotional, interpersonal and cultural resources to support them and to protect them against the effects of stress. Antonovsky described these as 'general resistance resources' which, when combined with a successful coping history, appeared to provide the individual with a personal 'sense of coherence'. Having a positive sense of coherence is reported to be associated with a personality orientation which includes confidence that one's environment is predictable and controllable and that coping resources are available to meet demands. People with a strong sense of coherence tend to view demands in terms of positive challenges worthy of engagement (Antonovsky 1987).

Relatives of patients dying in hospital may have their sense of coherence preserved or strengthened by care that is supportive and that reduces uncertainty and increases feelings of control.

Kobasa (1979) studied stress in American executives and, like Antonovsky, found that, although some people exhibited symptoms of ill-health when exposed to stress, others stayed well. Kobasa attributed this apparent resilience to 'personality hardiness', which he characterized as a clear sense of self, an understanding of one's personal values, goals and capabilities, social involvement and an internal locus of control. People with hardy personalities tend to view change as a normal part of life that offers opportunities for personal development (Leefarr and Cutler 1994).

People with an internal locus of control tend to view themselves as active agents who are self-directing and able to exercise some control over events. Conversely, those with an external locus of control believe events to be outside their control and see their fate as being largely determined by external forces (Rotter 1966). Locus of control orientation has been linked to information-seeking behaviour, in that those with an internal locus of control are more likely to seek information actively (Smith et al. 1987; Steptoe et al. 1991). It has already been established in the literature that relatives of dying patients who have unmet needs for information experience significant stress.

Notions of personal control and mastery are central to Antonovsky's 'sense of coherence', Kobasa's 'personality hardiness' and Rotter's 'locus of control'. Control and mastery appear to exert a positive influence on coping outcomes and, in salutogenic terms, result in reduced levels of psychological or physical ill-health arising from stressful encounters (Antonovsky 1987).

Such findings can add significantly to our understanding of stress and coping during terminal illness. By acknowledging the distress and vulnerability that terminal illness can generate, not just in the patient but in the family and professional carers, it should be possible by offering information, education and support to enhance personal control and mastery, and to decrease feelings of powerlessness and alienation (Steptoe et al. 1991).

Folkman and Lazarus caution against overzealous orientation towards personality constructs as predictors of coping (Folkman 1984).

They suggest that trait theories erroneously assume that people will behave consistently across a range of situations, whereas 'state' theories assume, again erroneously, that within particular situations different people can be expected to respond similarly. In reality such consistency is rarely revealed. Coping involves multiple tasks and an array of strategies operating within contexts that are reflexive, shifting and dynamic (Folkman 1984). Moreover, overzealous reliance on personality theories of stress might cause value judgements to be made about people based on quite narrow constructs. Similarly, when coping is explored from a situational perspective, as in some of the reported bereavement studies, there is a risk that normative values might be inappropriately applied (Parkes 1978; Worden 1983).

It would seem that there is no omni-competent set of coping strategies that can serve as a protection for all circumstances in life. Also, notions of personal mastery and control without regard to situations and relationships tend to be no more than cultural ideals. Pearlin and Schooler sum up the results of their major investigation into stress and coping thus:

> The magic wand does not appear in our results and this suggests that having a particular weapon in one's arsenal is less important than having a variety of weapons. Effective coping might depend not so much on 'what we do' as on 'how much we do'. The greater the scope and variety of resources in a person's coping repertoire the more protection coping affords.
>
> (Pearlin and Schooler 1978, p. 13)

Rationale for choice of framework

Wrubel and colleagues (1981) recommend that, when exploring aspects of stress and coping, one should search for neither determinant traits within the individual nor inescapable forces in the environment, but should look instead to the ways in which individuals and their social contexts mutually influence each other.

The holistic and humanistic orientation of the cognitive, phenomenological, transactional model of stress and coping, with its responsive and reflexive characteristics (Wrubel et al. 1981), appears to offer the most promising potential for enhanced understanding of the unique subjective experiences of dying patients' relatives and of the staff nurses who provide care. It also offers a coherent but sensitive thread to connect the myriad and complex contextual factors that operate within terminal care in hospital. Also, as the subjective experience of stress represents a common and unifying factor in this complex situation, this framework should allow the dual perspectives of caregivers and care recipients to be jointly explored.

For these reasons the cognitive, phenomenological, transactional model has been adopted as the theoretical framework for the current study. It is hoped that this approach might offer a path to discover the needs and concerns of the nurses and relatives, and that it will also offer a coherent yet sensitive framework within which to design and subsequently evaluate ways to support both relatives and nurses and to augment their repertoire of coping resources.

Chapter 4
Approach and methods

In this chapter the approach selected for the study is described and some of the methodological decisions that were taken during the course of the investigation explained. It should be stated at the outset that the philosophical and methodological basis of this study did not remain static throughout the course of the investigation, but rather developed and evolved in response to the dynamic and reflexive influences at work within the research environment.

In the early planning stages of the investigation, it was judged that the aims of the study would best be met by employing an evaluation research design, conducted within a quality assurance framework using a qualitative approach for data gathering and analysis. As is customary in such an approach, the literature was searched in order to establish current knowledge and to guide selection of the theoretical framework and development of the instruments. Before going on to report how these research methods were applied within the study, and to describe the philosophical shifts that occurred, the principles and main characteristics of evaluation research, quality assurance and qualitative research methodology are reviewed briefly.

Evaluation research

The term 'evaluation' is widely used to convey the notion of judgements about merit or worth. In this sense, evaluation does not presuppose a systematic process of enquiry or require presentation of objective evidence. On the other hand 'evaluation research' implies the use of scientific methods and techniques for the purpose of making judgements about the impact and effectiveness of a programme or practice. Wright (1989) accommodates differing interpretations of the term 'evaluation' and the range of activities that might be encompassed by placing these along a continuum, with value judgements occupying one end and rigorous research methodology the other.

Evaluation research covers a range of investigative and problem-solving activities aimed at judging the merit or worth of a programme or practice (Powers and Knapp 1995). Together with needs analysis and action research, evaluation research represents one of a cluster of research types collectively classified as applied research (Tesch 1990). Applied research is essentially improvement oriented because it seeks to use the knowledge generated in an investigation to develop solutions to practical problems. In this respect, applied research can be contrasted with basic research where the sole aim is the generation of knowledge (Powers and Knapp 1995).

Marsland and Gissane (1992) trace the origins of evaluation research to large-scale educational programmes mainly funded by governments. Historically, this was most evident in the USA, where laws were passed during the 1960s to ensure that programmes supported by public investments incorporated mechanisms for systematic evaluation (Marsland and Gissane 1992). From these beginnings, evaluation research expanded into a large-scale discipline which, although still strongly grounded within the field of education, has spread to other areas including health care. Indeed, under the auspices of bodies such as the World Health Organization (WHO), worldwide health programmes are now the subject of systematic evaluation research (Marsland and Gissane 1992).

In evaluation research, the focus tends to be on the measurement of change, and the approach commonly requires judgements to be made within an 'action setting'. Luker (1981) argues that constraints imposed by an action setting do not change the methodological duties of the investigator. While recommending the randomized controlled experiment as the 'ideal' design, Luker (1981) acknowledges that within social situations ethical and practical difficulties often preclude the use of the experimental approach. In response to such practical and ethical concerns, a range of models and approaches to evaluation research was developed.

Classification and models

Evaluation research can be classified in various ways. A commonly used classification relates to the philosophical origins of the approach and, in common with other research methods, evaluation research is broadly classified as qualitative or quantitative according to the approach used and techniques applied during data gathering and analysis (Gallego 1987). Gallego contrasts quantitative and qualitative evaluation research models by placing their key features along a number of continua. Gallego's analysis reveals that quantitative evaluation research models are characterized by strict methodological control and objectivity, with a primary focus on establishing causality when evaluating the outcomes of a programme or practice (Gallego 1987). In qualitative evaluation research, methodological control is more problematic, the knowledge generated is more subjective, albeit more applicable, and the evaluation focus is on the processes that occur within a programme rather than being solely based on measurable outcomes (Gallego 1987).

An alternative approach to classifying evaluation research models considers the extent to which evaluation processes rely on pre-specified criteria or objectives, e.g. the 'Goal Attainment Model' typically employs experimental or quasi-experimental methods such as pre-test post-test design and evaluates outcomes in relation to predetermined objectives or criteria (Suchman 1967). In contrast, the 'Goal Free' approach employs mainly qualitative approaches and usually incorporates the participants' subjective judgements in the overall evaluations. The goal-free approach also acknowledges the complex interactive processes at work within an action setting (Polit and Hungler 1991). The illuminative model of evaluation (Parlett and Hamilton 1972) represents a goal-free approach that seeks to make evaluation more holistic and responsive to influences that occur within an action setting.

Lattimer (1991) suggests that, historically, the goal-free or illuminative approach to evaluation developed from the evaluation researchers' ongoing struggle to reconcile the competing demands for scientific purity of research method with the need for utility of evaluation findings. Illuminative evaluation focuses on process rather than adopting a single focus on programme outcomes and incorporates qualitative methods for data gathering and analysis. In the illuminative approach to evaluation, data are often drawn from a range of sources and seek multiple perspectives which often include the consumers' views about a programme or practice. In recognition of the dynamic properties of most action settings, illuminative evaluation tends to be highly reflexive and reflective in character (Gallego 1987). Lattimer (1991) argues that the illuminative evaluator should seek to expose subjective elements in the evaluation, and present an account of the research process that allows the quality of the findings to be fully judged.

This move away from insistence on the experimental or quasi-experimental approach towards a more open acceptance of qualitative approaches in evaluation research represents a paradigm shift away from the monolithic approach towards a more pluralistic and holistic conception of evaluation (House 1993). Philosophically, evaluators have now ceased to believe their discipline to be value free, and traditional notions of external and internal validity in evaluation research have been challenged. Evaluation research now commonly utilizes complex processes that might incorporate multiple measures, methods, criteria and perspectives (House 1993).

Quality assurance and evaluation

Although the literature on evaluation research is heavily weighted towards educational evaluation, health-care *practice* evaluation programmes are commonly conducted within a quality assurance framework (Luker 1981; Wright 1989; Powers and Knapp 1995). Quality assurance methods involve the planned and systematic use of selected evaluation tools designed to measure pre-specified criteria against agreed standards. Quality assurance also involves the institution of corrective actions needed to achieve and maintain quality in health care, and in this respect this approach is seen as more proactive than other evaluation models which tend to be retrospective in focus.

Donabedian, a physician, prolific writer and pioneer in evaluation research in health care, developed an influential model for designing, implementing and evaluating quality improvement programmes in the field of health using a quality assurance framework (Luker 1981). Donabedian's approach represents a 'Goal Attainment' model in that achievement of pre-specified standard criteria are measured, typically using audit techniques. Quality assurance audit processes facilitate formative evaluation by providing feedback to practitioners, to enable adjustments to be made to interventions; it can also contribute to summative evaluation, enabling the overall impact of an intervention to be assessed (Donabedian 1988).

Approaches to setting of standards

The very act of standard setting is often enough to signal the beginning of improved care because the process can act as a catalyst for change and can empower people as they work towards changing their practice (Methot, Caesar and Duquette 1992). Approaches to standard setting have been described alternatively as 'top down' or 'bottom up' (Poulton 1992). In the top-down approach, managers or researchers decide which aspects of practice need to be improved and how these changes should be achieved, and a standard is then provided for the care team to work to. Evidence suggests that standards imposed from 'above' in this way may fail to be adopted because of a lack of commitment and of feelings of ownership on the part of practitioners (Sale 1988; Garvey and Manley 1992; Mackenzie 1992; Kitson 1993). Moreover, uniform standards, especially of the top-down variety, can represent the antithesis of individualized care as a result of their tendency to itemize and decontextualize nursing care (Cheddel 1991).

In the 'bottom-up' approach, those who deliver the care are closely involved in the design, implementation and evaluation processes (Harvey 1988a). The 'Dynamic Standard Setting System' (DySSSy) represents one such approach. The key stages include: writing and implementing a standard; developing an audit tool to monitor its effect; collecting and collating audit data; and implementing appropriate action for quality improvement (Poulton 1992; Harvey 1994; Gibson 1995). The DySSSy approach utilizes the Donabedian evaluation model (Donabedian 1988). A standard statement is developed which encapsulates the agreed standard of care and structure, process and outcome criteria are then specified. 'Structure' criteria include resources such as money, buildings, facilities, equipment and the human resources needed to achieve the agreed standard. 'Process' criteria represent procedures and actions involved in meeting the standard, whereas 'outcome' criteria detail, in measurable terms, the required results (Poulton 1992; Kitson 1993; Harvey 1994; Gibson 1995).

Using the DySSSy approach to standard setting, the Royal College of Nursing (1991) produced core standards for aspects of cancer nursing, including terminal care, and the Trent Hospice and Audit Group implemented and evaluated a standard-setting initiative within a number of hospice settings (Ingleton and Faulkner 1993). Evaluation data from the Trent initiative revealed that staff often experience difficulties with the process of developing standards. The authors recommend providing an education programme before embarking on a standard-setting initiative and they firmly endorse the 'bottom-up' approach, which devolves ownership and control to practitioners (Ingleton and Faulkner 1993). Ingleton and Faulkner's views are supported by Kitson (1986) who further argues that the success of a standard-setting initiative will be significantly increased by having an experienced facilitator who can provide information, feedback and support to the standard-setting group.

The current study seeks to address both of these recommendations by providing an educational initiative in the form of a workshop and by offering ongoing support from the researcher as the nurses work towards implementing their standards in their own wards.

Auditing standards of care

Standard setting encourages practitioners to reflect upon and evaluate their practice (Koch 1992). Audit represents part of the quality assurance cycle, and involves systematic and critical analysis of resources, activities, practices and outcomes. Audit approaches might include asking people's views, observing and measuring specific outcomes, and checking records and charts (Koch 1992). A number of validated audit tools exist such as 'Qualpacs' or 'Monitor' to record audit data (Harvey 1988a, 1988b). These tools reveal a strong quantitative slant mainly using numerical scores to record and measure quality of care.

Koch (1992) argues that an evaluation approach that relies solely on numerical measurement in the form of audit data, and that reports in terms that are 'unilateral and brook no dissent', allows experts to determine what constitutes quality while patients and clients are unable to enter the evaluation debate. Koch recommends an illuminative approach to evaluating quality initiatives and, in particular, advocates qualitative methods that involve communicating directly with patients and clients to elicit their views and concerns, arguing that such methods have the potential to improve nurses' understanding of what it 'means' to be a patient (Koch 1992). Mackenzie (1992) concurs with this view, also advocating clear, research-based standards that use the views of the consumer.

Selection of evaluation model

Experimental or quasi-experimental evaluation approaches such as pre- and post-test design, which require examination of causality between selected independent and dependent variables, were judged to be inappropriate for the current study because it was unclear at the outset what the goals would be or, indeed, whether these would be consistent across the different locations. For these reasons, a quality assurance model combined with qualitative approaches for gathering and analysing pre- and post-intervention interview data was selected as the evaluation design for the study.

Donabedian's quality assurance framework was selected for implementing and evaluating the planned intervention in the current study because it was judged likely that the participating nurses and their ward teams would be familiar with this established approach to standard setting. It was further judged that a standard-setting approach would allow the intervention to be designed by those most directly responsible for its implementation. It has already been established that such involvement of practitioners is an important factor in promoting a sense of ownership of and commitment to an improvement initiative (Kitson 1986; Harvey 1994). Finally, standard setting was favoured as the approach that encourages nurses to engage in reflection on and evaluation of their own practice (Methot et al. 1992). A quality assurance framework also facilitates formative evaluation, thus allowing practitioners to take corrective actions to ensure quality of care.

To counterbalance the quantitative slant characteristic of quality assurance evaluation strategies, a number of authors recommend incorporating qualitative approaches that seek the consumers' feelings and concerns (Koch 1992; Ingleton and Faulkner 1993; Kitson 1993). Within the current study, it was judged that the change initiative could be viewed in its fullest possible context by using pre- and post-intervention qualitative research data from both practitioners and consumers in the design, implementation and evaluation of changes in practice. For these reasons an evaluation strategy that incorporated the dual perspectives of practitioners and consumers, and also combined quality assurance data with qualitative interview data in the evaluation process, was selected.

Evaluation research is essentially retrospective in its gaze because the method seeks to discern patterns of deficiency by reflecting on aspects of a programme after the events have taken place. The evaluation researcher's role is to gather and analyse data and, although this can involve multiple methods and data sources, the researcher usually remains separate from the events that are occurring in the action setting during the course of the change initiative.

It is revealed in Chapter 6 that, during the course of the extended intervention period, the character of the current investigation changed in response to a range of reflexive influences that were occurring within the research environment. During this period of intensive activity, the participants' level of involvement in the research process increased sharply and the distance between the researcher and the participants decreased correspondingly. The effects of these changed study dynamics caused the relatively passive evaluation research design to develop into a participative and collaborative endeavour, within which the researcher adopted the role of supporter to the participating nurses in their role as an agent for change. As a result of these changes the research method became more consistent with the action research approach.

The main characteristics that distinguish action research from evaluation research are the level of involvement of practitioners in the research activities and the distance that operates within the researcher–participant relationship. Action research seeks to overcome the passivity of other research methods in that the researcher–participant relationship is essentially collaborative and research participants become stakeholders in studies that are, in turn, responsive to their own interests and practical concerns (Tesch 1990; Waddell 1991; Powers and Knapp 1995). An account of the methodological shift that occurred, and the associated literature on

planned change and action research, is more fully reported in
Chapter 6 because this represents an accurate account of the study
activities.

Qualitative research

The 'paradigm wars' described by Guba and Lincoln (1994) consti-
tute the often heated debate about the relative merits of quantitative
(positivist) and qualitative (naturalist) methods of enquiry. The divide
that separates the major research paradigms has, to some extent,
already been underlined earlier in this chapter, during the course of
examining different models of evaluation research.

Quantitative methods based on measurement, deductive reasoning, causality and hypothesis testing are traditionally viewed as
'scientific' and objective in character. Quantitative studies typically
have a well-circumscribed focus of enquiry, sample sizes tend to be
large and the numerical data generated in the study can be subjected
to statistical testing. Accordingly, claims are made for the predictive
powers of quantitative methods and the generalizability of their findings. Positivist methods have, however, also been described as reductionist as a result of their tendency to study phenomena stripped of
their context (Leininger 1984; Clarke 1991).

Historically nurse researchers, in their desire for professional
respectability, have tended to employ mainly positivist methods in
their investigations (Melia 1982). Although the scientific method is
entirely appropriate in many areas of study, Leonard (1989) recommends that it should be confined to investigations 'where the participants' meanings and interpretations don't figure'. This view is
echoed by Clarke (1991) who argues forcefully that in health-care
research 'the tendency to apply positivist criteria to the study of
human action has resulted in grotesque parodies which have almost
completely crippled our quest for understanding'.

In qualitative (naturalist) methods, phenomena are studied within
their natural setting with the aim of bringing the respondents'
subjective experience to light. It has been suggested that appropriate
use of qualitative methods can help to close the gap between discovery and implementation, and can lead to a deeper understanding of
the many and complex phenomena intrinsic to health-care investigations (Joni 1995).

The main qualitative approaches include ethnography, grounded theory and phenomenology. Although these approaches show many commonalities, especially in relation to the centrality that each affords to subjective experience and to the multiple realities that exist within any phenomenon, each tradition has different roots and their philosophies and methodologies differ.

Ethnography has its roots in anthropology and the aim of the method is to render one 'culture' understandable to another. Ethnographic studies typically require extended periods of field work and use observation and interview methods for data gathering. The investigator enters the field with an 'etic' (outsider's) view and sets out to achieve an 'emic' (insider's) perspective (Leininger 1984). Leininger uses the 'back-stage/front-stage' concept to illustrate the importance of gaining the trust and acceptance of those being studied. In the early stages of a research relationship the actors (participants) and the researcher remain front stage where the investigator is treated with caution and the emerging data can be sparse and unreliable. Acceptance and trust enable a more intimate relationship to develop and allow the actor and the now researcher–friend to move back stage to where the data are more copious, rich and reliable (Leininger 1984).

Thorne (1991) suggests that nurse researchers rarely conduct whole ethnographies. More typically they borrow ethnographic methods to study discrete aspects of health-related behaviours. Used in this way, ethnographic methods have provided insight into particular client groups and their concerns (Leininger 1984; Sandelowski 1991; Mackenzie 1994).

Grounded theory represents another major branch of qualitative research. It has its roots in certain sociological theories and, in particular, in symbolic interactionism where the focus of interest is the symbolic meanings that people attribute to the events and transactions in their lives, and on the ways people interact within their social roles (Glaser and Strauss 1967; Blumer 1969; Bowers 1992). In the grounded theory method, observation and interview data are collected within their natural setting and analysis processes generate codes, categories and substantive theory. Data gathering and analysis occur simultaneously and are terminated when inductively based theories emerge that adequately explain the situation under study (Glaser and Strauss 1967; Wilson and Hutchieson 1991; Wainwright 1994).

Phenomenology is both a philosophy and a research method. It holds considerable appeal for disciplines such as philosophy, psychology, and nursing which share its concern for the unique quality of each human being and the need to understand the 'lived' experience of others (Thorne 1991). Phenomenology offers a radical departure from the Cartesian, biomedical, positivist view of the person as an assemblage of traits or symptoms that can be studied in isolation from their wider context (Leonard 1989; Walters 1994).

Much current phenomenological thinking stems from the works of Husserl, a late nineteenth century philosopher (Reeder 1987). The philosophical underpinnings are complex and focus on essential questions of epistemology (the nature of knowing) and ontology (the nature of being). In phenomenology, the epistemological position is that basic human truths are accessible only through subjectivity and by searching beneath the assumptions of the sciences to expose the roots of the lived experience (Thorne 1991).

Heidegger, a student of Husserl, developed a branch of phenomenology known as hermeneutics. Heidegger, like Husserl, acknowledged the centrality of the subjective experience, but he rejected Husserl's notion of the person as a private and disconnected being who merely responds to an objective world (Benner 1985). Heideggerian thinking holds that each person's 'world' is constructed from the common and shared understandings that make up his or her 'being-in-the-world'. A person's world can therefore be understood only when viewed within the context of his or her relationships, background, culture and language (Reeder 1987; Darbyshire 1992).

Heideggerian phenomenology and nursing share a common concern for the subjective reality of experiences and for the moral value of interacting with each person as a unique being deserving of equally unique caring interventions (Benner 1983; Thorne 1991). Indeed, according to Leininger (1984), when nurses empathize with and attempt to understand individual clients, they bring a phenomenological attitude to their practice. Walters also suggests that, when nurses practise in a phenomenological way, they can transcend the Cartesian perspective characterized by the medical model to focus on each patient's unique lived experience, and in this way the technological reality of health care can be rendered transparent to allow the humanistic dimension of care to shine through (Walters 1994).

Selection of qualitative framework

As the present study was not directly concerned with interpreting culture, and as the single interview contact with the relatives did not satisfy the criteria normally associated with ethnographic methods, this approach did not seem to meet the requirements of the study. If the focus of the study had been in an area about which little was currently known, grounded theory might have offered an appropriate choice. However, by the time the current study was embarked upon the researcher already had considerable professional experience in the area and had gained further insights from the literature. For these reasons the grounded theory method was also rejected.

Phenomenology would undoubtedly have offered the most appropriate approach if the intention had been to explore and illuminate the lived experience as an end in itself. However, the purpose of the current study was to generate data that would be used to develop, implement and evaluate an intervention. Moreover, factors such as the initial choice of evaluation research design, the fairly structured instruments and the decision to work within a theoretical framework, together with the data yield anticipated from about 80 in-depth interviews, did not appear to be congruent with the ethos and philosophy associated with the phenomenological tradition. Accordingly, this path to data gathering and analysis was not initially taken, although this decision was reviewed at a later stage in the investigation.

This brief examination of the potential utility of the main qualitative approaches revealed that, in their 'pure' sense, none precisely met the needs of the current study. Each tradition was developed to serve the specific disciplines of sociology, anthropology and philosophy and, for the most part, the focus of their research is to generate knowledge. In contrast researchers in practice disciplines such as nursing often have to meet the dual demands of knowledge generation and practical utility in their research endeavours. When conducting applied research, investigators have often to adapt their method to accommodate dynamic and reflexive influences that occur within a practice setting. For these reasons, nurse researchers commonly experience difficulty in expressing a specific allegiance to one of the main qualitative traditions (Thorne 1991; Sandelowski 1993a).

It should be noted that, within the current study, the term 'reflexivity' is used to describe the dynamic and reciprocal relationships that occur within the research environment and the influence that such factors have on the overall conduct of the investigation (Lamb and Huttlinger 1991).

The rising interest in human science research approaches and the trend towards convergence between disciplines within the social sciences has led to a greater acceptance of broad social science approaches being used within an applied research framework. Such methods, although qualitative in respect of the techniques employed, are not necessarily committed to one particular qualitative research tradition (Powers and Knapp 1995). The growing tendency towards methodological eclecticism was underscored by Tesch (1990) who identified and classified 26 recorded varieties of qualitative research. Tesch used the painter's palette as a metaphor to illustrate the range and diversity of recorded qualitative approaches, suggesting that the main qualitative traditions are represented by the basic colours that can be mixed to produce an unending variety of shades. She argues that, although maintaining fidelity to the spirit of the qualitative tradition, each researcher might have to create her or his own unique shade. Tesch concludes her discourse thus:

> Just because some investigator has given her particular 'shade' a name and has written about it doesn't mean that it must be used in exactly that way for ever more – always keeping each of its tenets intact. To be sure, some types of research, and some labels, catch on more strongly, or have a longer tradition than others. But basically there is but one requirement from research: that you can persuade others that you have indeed made a discovery worthy of paying attention to.
>
> (Tesch 1990, p. 71)

Although employing a quality assurance framework for implementing and evaluating the planned change initiative, an eclectic approach to gathering and analysing the pre- and post-intervention qualitative interview data was initially adopted for the current study. During the course of the study, the researcher's philosophical orientation shifted in response to influences that occurred during the processes of data analysis. These events are reported later in the chapter.

The pilot study

To test the approach and methods and the analysis techniques, a pilot study was conducted during which five relatives and five staff nurses were interviewed and the resulting data analysed.

The interview approach

A semi-structured interview approach was selected using mainly open questions designed to elicit the participants' perceptions, feelings and concerns. It was judged that such an approach would allow themes that had emerged from the literature to be pursued and would enable the theoretical framework to be incorporated, by including questions that explored the nature of the stress experienced and the range of coping strategies employed by the relatives and the nurses. Data emerging from analysis of the relatives' and nurses' interviews would then be used to develop and implement an intervention aimed at improving family support in each of the study wards.

The decision to adopt a semi-structured interview approach for gathering pre- and post-intervention data was taken because it was judged that a questionnaire might prove too restrictive when exploring the experiences, feelings and attitudes of the respondents in such a sensitive area of study. Also, the interview approach was favoured because it allows the interviewer to pursue themes and to offer and seek clarification during the course of the encounter. Interviews also provide the potential to get beyond a surface understanding of the phenomena being studied and the approach accommodates the interactive nature of relationships that operate between the researcher and the study participants (Kvale 1983; Sandelowski et al. 1989; Corner 1991b; Lamb and Huttlinger 1991; Guba and Lincoln 1994).

The pilot study also enabled testing of the approach for gaining access to the relatives' sample. The sampling strategy adopted, fully described in the next section, was found to be acceptable to the relatives. The instruments were also tested and minor adjustments made to the relatives' interview schedule after the pilot study, e.g. an unanticipated issue that was raised by relatives in the pilot study related to the potential economic impact that protracted illness can have on the family. Accordingly an additional question was inserted to ensure that this issue was explored with relatives during the main study interviews. Also a slight reordering of questions was undertaken to improve the flow of the dialogue. Overall the instruments proved to be effective in that they yielded copious rich data, and the question style and delivery were reported as acceptable by the interviewees.

Pilot study analysis

Attention is drawn to the procedural aspects of data analysis at this point because the analysis approach was changed during the course of the pilot study.

The interviews were transcribed in full and a line-by-line analysis of the hard copies of the transcribed text was conducted. From those analysis processes, categorizing and coding frameworks were developed for both the nurses' and the relatives' data.

The relatives' data were much richer and more detailed than had been expected. Their need to express the powerful emotions bound up in this sensitive situation, the complexity of their experiences, and their need to place these experiences in context by reflecting right back from the time of the diagnosis to the present time were evident.

The nurses' data similarly revealed their need to express the nature and the degree of stress that they experienced with this aspect of their role, their views about their professional preparation in this area, and their access to support and continuing education in this field.

As a result of the volume and richness of these pilot data, and the concerns raised about managing the much greater volume of data anticipated in the main study, the potential merit of employing a computerized approach to analysis was investigated. Accordingly, data from the pilot interviews were analysed for a second time using Hyperqual2.1, a qualitative textual analysis package designed for the Macintosh computer (Padilla 1993).

Computerized analysis

Hyperqual2.1 was selected because this package offered the capability of searching, sorting, linking and printing data both within a data set and between different data sets. A practical advantage of this programme was that raw data could be transcribed directly into the software, thus avoiding the need to import transcribed text from the word processor. Hyperqual employs the principle of index cards to store, manipulate and retrieve data. A single card may contain up to 30 000 characters and each card has a unique identity number. Within the program, cards are organized into stacks that can be of various types.

The pilot data were first entered into two separate 'interview data' stacks: one for the nurses and the other for the relatives. Within each interview data stack, every respondent has a 'personal face card', containing biographical and other details about that person. This is followed by a series of 'data cards' each containing that respondent's answer to an individual question. This arrangement of a face card followed by a series of data cards was repeated, until all of the audio-tapes from that particular sample had been transcribed.

During the processes of analysis, themes emerged and data that focused on the emerging themes were identified, tagged and exported to form new homogeneous stacks. Iterative processes of sorting, grouping and ultimately printing related data in this way allowed commonalities and uniqueness in the accounts to be explored. Navigation both within and between stacks was possible using the electronic linkages provided by the program. This ensured that segments of text could have their context retained. Comparison of the results achieved from the manual and electronic analysis approaches provided convincing evidence that depth and rigour of analysis were enhanced by using the software and confirmed the decision that this would be the strategy of choice for the main study.

The above is included at this stage to offer a description of the structural and operational characteristics of the software and, in so doing, to demonstrate the utility of this particular approach. The cognitive and interpretative aspects of this form of analysis are explored in more detail during the description of the main study analysis on pages 82–89.

The main study

Aims of the study

- To explore and describe the needs and concerns of relatives of dying cancer patients in acute hospital wards and the concerns of nurses involved in providing care.

- To use these data to design, implement and evaluate quality assurance standards for improved care and support of families during terminal illness.

Study objectives

The study seeks to:

1. Elicit from relatives of terminally ill cancer patients in acute hospital wards:
   - their perceived needs for care and support from nurses
   - the extent to which those needs are currently being met
   - the stress that they experience in relation to unmet needs
   - the coping strategies that they employ.
2. Elicit from staff nurses who provide terminal care in acute hospital wards:
   - their perceptions of the needs of relatives of dying patients
   - the extent to which they believe these needs are being met
   - their concerns and difficulties in relation to this aspect of care
   - the coping strategies that they employ.
3. Utilize the research data provided by the relatives and the staff nurses to:
   - design quality assurance standards for improved care and support of relatives of dying patients
   - implement the standards in the designated study wards
   - evaluate the extent to which the standard criteria have been met.

After a designated period, during which the standards are implemented and evaluated within given clinical settings:

4. Elicit from a *second* sample of relatives:
   - their perceived needs for care and support from nurses
   - the extent to which those needs are currently being met.
5. Elicit from *the same sample* of staff nurses:
   - the extent to which the nurses believe that the relatives' needs are currently being met
   - the nature and degree of stress currently associated with this aspect of their practice.

Definition of terms

For the purposes of the proposed study, the following definitions apply.

Terminally ill patients

This includes adult hospitalized patients with advanced malignant disease for whom the entire focus of care is palliative. The patients have been diagnosed by their physician as being in the advanced stages of terminal illness and unlikely to be discharged from hospital before death.

Acute hospital setting

The study setting includes acute medical and surgical wards in two major teaching hospitals. Specialist areas such as oncology wards or palliative care settings are not included.

Relatives

This term encompasses those people who are judged by the nurses who are caring for the patient to have the closest emotional bond with the patient. It is likely that this mainly (but not exclusively) includes people who have close kinship ties with the patient. Also, the person identified as 'closest to the patient' need not be the person recorded in the admission documents as the patient's legal next of kin. Only people aged 18 years or over are included in the relatives' sample.

Design overview

The study design had two phases separated by an intervention. During the course of the study three samples were recruited, one of staff nurses and two of relatives. One of the relatives' samples was recruited during phase 1 of the study and the other during phase 2. During phase 1, interviews were conducted with the staff nurses and the first sample of relatives, to elicit their needs and concerns. During the intervention period that followed, the nurses attended a 2-day workshop, where they used data from the phase 1 analysis to design quality assurance standards for improved family support during terminal illness. The staff nurses then acted as facilitators as the standards were implemented and evaluated in their own wards. During phase 2, a second sample of relatives was recruited and interviewed, and the nurses had a second short interview. Comparative analysis of the phase 1 and phase 2 data contributed to the final evaluation of the intervention.

The setting

The study was conducted in eight acute wards in two large city hospitals in Scotland. Acute wards were selected because, despite the increased numbers of hospice and home deaths, most cancer patients still die in hospital wards (Greater Glasgow Health Board 1995). Within each hospital, two medical and two surgical wards were selected. When selecting wards for inclusion, advice was sought from nurse managers about wards that, although not designated as 'specialist' palliative care or oncology wards, regularly provide care for dying cancer patients and their families. The decision to focus on 'general' wards was taken because it was judged that nurses in nonspecialist areas might have had fewer opportunities to acquire specific expertise or training in relation to this aspect of care, and that their needs and concerns, and those of dying patients' relatives in these wards, might merit particular investigation.

Access negotiations

With the permission of the Chief Area Nursing Officer (CANO), the Director of Nursing Service (DNS) for each hospital was approached to request access for the study and both gave their permission. In hospital A, the researcher was invited to a meeting with the senior nurse managers to explain the aims and scope of the study and to identify suitable wards for inclusion in the study. In hospital B, the DNS identified wards for inclusion and the researcher contacted the relevant managers before contacting the ward sisters/charge nurses. Subsequently, meetings were arranged with each of the ward sisters/charge nurses on both sites to provide information about the study and to seek permission to use their ward as a study site. All of the ward sisters/charge nurses who were approached agreed to have their ward included. A folder containing information about the study was provided for each ward.

Medical consultants and clinical directors were contacted by letter to seek access to the proposed study wards. An outline of the study design and the ethical approval documents were enclosed with the letter. Although it took quite some time to complete this process, permission for access was eventually given by all of the clinical directors and consultants.

Samples and methods

In the following section, the procedures adopted for gaining the relatives' and nurses' samples are detailed and the main characteristics of each sample described. The approach used for analysing and interpreting the interview data is also detailed. A decision was taken to devote a specific chapter (Chapter 6) to describing the intervention and associated literature because this represents a complex and crucially important part of the current study. This also enables the report on the intervention to be located at its logical, chronological place – namely after discussion of the phase 1 results and preceding the report on phase 2 of the study.

The relatives

Acquiring the relatives' samples

The samples include the 'closest relatives' of patients with terminal carcinoma, in the final weeks of their illness, receiving care that is purely palliative and unlikely to be discharged home. As stated earlier in this chapter, the relative need not necessarily be 'related' by kinship to the patient. Cancer patients' relatives were selected because it was felt that they might have had common experiences in terms of the impact of the diagnosis on the family, the effects of the patient's symptoms and of the various forms of cancer treatment, and having to face the implications of a shift to a purely palliative mode of treatment (Lewis 1986). Such a shift in focus may not be seen so explicitly in other disease groups, such as patients with cardiovascular or respiratory disorders.

Selection of the closest relative was based on the nurses' knowledge of kinship or other close emotional ties, and the frequency of visiting and contact. The closest relative may, but need not necessarily, be recorded as next of kin in the patient's notes. A card detailing the sample inclusion criteria and guidelines about how the relatives should be approached was placed in the 'research study folder' in the wards.

As the family is likely to be under considerable stress at this time, the decision to include just one adult relative for each dying patient was taken. The participating nurses were responsible for identifying relatives who met the inclusion criteria and for offering the relative a letter from the researcher. The letter provided background information about the researcher, outlined the main aim of the study and sought permission for the researcher to make contact with the relative. The relatives selected whether or not contact could be made by the researcher and, if an initial contact was agreed to, whether this should be by telephone or by meeting them in person at the ward.

During this preliminary contact, the relative and researcher were able to communicate directly, further information about the study was provided and relatives were asked whether they would be willing to be interviewed. For those who consented to be interviewed, and this represented every relative who had agreed to the initial contact from the researcher, a date, time and location for the interview were agreed. Relatives were informed of their right to withdraw from the study at any stage should they wish to do so and assured that their rights to confidentiality would be observed.

The phase 1 relatives

During phase 1 of the study, 35 relatives were approached and offered a letter. Six patients died much sooner than predicted and before an interview could take place. From a possible sample of 29 relatives, 23 agreed to the initial approach by the researcher and all 23 subsequently agreed to be interviewed, resulting in an 'opt-in' rate of 79%. In keeping with the design of the study, three relatives had a second interview 2 weeks after the first because their loved one was still in the ward at that time. A second interview was offered to try to capture the dynamic character of the relatives' experiences during the time leading up to their loved one's death, and also to avoid the situation in which the newly established researcher–relative contact was abruptly severed.

A total of 26 phase 1 relatives' interviews were conducted, 23 first interviews and 3 second interviews. These interviews lasted between 20 and 95 min (mean = 55 min).

Sample profile (Table 4.1)

The relatives' ages ranged from 32 to 70 years (mean = 58 years). The sample contained 20 women and 3 men and represented a range of relationships. The patients' ages ranged from 55 to 82 years (mean = 69 years). The relatives' perceptions of the diagnosis revealed a range of tumour sites.

Table 4.1: Sample profile for phase 1 relatives

Length of interviews	20 min to 95 min (mean = 55 min)	
Relatives' ages	32–70 years (mean = 58 years)	
Sex distribution	20 female and 3 male	
Range of relationships	9 daughters	1 son
	6 wives	2 husbands
	1 sister	1 sister-in-law
	1 niece	2 close friends
Patients' age range	55–82 years (mean = 69 years)	
Patients' diagnosis	Primary tumour sites	
	Lung 12	Oesophagus 3
	Stomach/bowel 3	Breast 1
	Abdominal mass 1	Cervix 1
	Prostate 1	Myeloma 1

The phase 2 relatives

Thirty-four letters were distributed during phase 2 of the study. One relative refused the introductory letter and four used the return slip to decline to be interviewed (one of whom sent her apologies and her best wishes for the study). In one family, where literacy difficulties were suspected, the letter was returned blank. Two patients went home, one was transferred to a hospice and seven died before an interview could be arranged with the relative. Twenty-two relatives' interviews were conducted during phase 2 of the study: 21 first interviews and 1 second interview.

Sample profile

The phase 2 relatives' interviews lasted between 40 and 65 min (mean = 49 min). Relatives' ages ranged from 42 to 73 years (mean = 54 years). The sample contained 16 women and 5 men, and a range of relationships was represented. The patients' ages ranged from 39 to 90 years (mean = 72 years). The relatives' perceptions of their loved one's diagnosis revealed that, although most of the patients had widespread metastasis, a wide range of primary tumour sites was reported. The main characteristics of both relatives' samples and the patients' diagnosis are summarized in Table 4.2.

Table 4.2: Sample profile for phase 2 relatives

Length of interview	40 min to 65 min (mean = 49 min)		
Relatives' ages	42–73 years (mean = 54 years)		
Sex distribution	16 female and 5 male		
Range of relationships	6 wives		
	2 husbands		
	9 daughters		
	1 daughter-in-law		
	3 sons		
Patients' age range	39–90 years (mean = 72 years)		
Patients' diagnosis	Primary tumour sites		
	Ovary	2	Vulva	1
	Prostate	1	Renal	1
	Breast	1	Lung	7
	Colon	2	Oesophagus	2
	Abdomen	2	Liver	2

Sampling issues

As qualitative investigations rely on the willing cooperation of participants who are prepared to share their particular experiences, convenience or purposive sampling methods are the most common (Bowling 1991; Hek 1995). Convenience samples include subjects who are available and willing to participate. In purposive sampling, the researcher defines specific inclusion and exclusion criteria based on knowledge of the phenomena to be studied. In either event, it is often the most articulate who are represented. Relatives recruited into the current study almost certainly represented people whom the nurses felt comfortable about approaching. Although it is understandable that nurses might feel hesitant about approaching angry or uncooperative relatives, the possibility of élite bias must therefore be acknowledged.

The nurses admit to having exercised judgement about whether an approach might cause unacceptable distress to the relatives or to themselves. Comments were made about some families whose distress was such that the nurses did not feel that the relatives could cope with an interview that focused on the source of their distress. The nurses' judgement in these matters had to be respected and the resulting sampling bias acknowledged.

Although working within the sample inclusion criteria, the decision about the precise point at which to offer relatives a letter rested with the nurses. It was commonly reported that patients had either died within a few days of admission, or that their condition had deteriorated so rapidly that the nurses were unable sensitively to offer a letter to the family. On other occasions, a letter was offered but there was inadequate time for the relatives to respond or for an interview to take place before the patient's death. Also, the reality of the situation militated against achieving matched samples of relatives in each phase of the study in terms of age, sex, diagnosis and relationship. However, the same interviewer, approach and instrument were used. The findings of the current study are interpreted with these potential limitations fully acknowledged.

The relatives' interviews

The instrument

The interview schedule, used with both samples of relatives, contained mainly open questions that were designed to explore the relatives' experiences, feelings and concerns. The design of the instrument was informed by themes derived from the literature and by the researcher's professional experience. The theoretical framework was incorporated using questions designed to elicit the nature of the relatives' stress and the coping strategies that they employed.

Themes explored during the relatives' interviews

- Pre-admission experiences
- Reasons for and response to admission
- Ward environment and facilities
- Emotional climate and staff–relative interface
- Information needs and access
- Relatives' stress (physical, psychological and socioeconomic)
- Coping strategies (usual and current)
- Support needs.

The interview approach

As has been previously reported, all of the relatives who agreed to the initial contact with the researcher subsequently agreed to be interviewed. Approximately half of the relatives chose to be interviewed at home and the other half elected to be interviewed in the ward while visiting their loved one. The researcher's preference was for home interviews, where the relatives were in their own familiar territory and could possibly feel more in control of the situation. In the home situation, the researcher also felt relieved of the concern that the interview might be taking the relative away from the loved one's bedside. It should be stated, however, that, when interviews were conducted within the hospital setting, relatives on the whole seemed to welcome the break from the bedside.

As previously reported, the pilot study had allowed adjustments to be made to the instrument so that a smooth conversational flow could be achieved. With experience, the researcher's interviewing technique became relaxed, refined and productive. Rather than being used as a rigid structure, the interview schedule then represented a flexible framework that was used for exploring salient themes. As the relatives had little difficulty in sustaining a steady flow of dialogue, the probes were infrequently used. Given that before the interview the relatives had met the researcher just once, and in many cases had only spoken with her on the phone, the depth, volume and richness of the data that emerged from the interviews were both surprising and gratifying.

The interviews were often emotionally charged encounters during which the researcher developed a bond with the relatives. On the return car journey from the interview, the tape recording was played for the first time. At this point the interviewer still felt somewhat emotionally connected to the respondent and could detect and appreciate nuances in the dialogue. On return to the home/office the tape was again played in full and brief notes were made. Conducting the interview, then listening to the tape immediately afterwards, and again within 1 or 2 hours of the interview, thoroughly captured the essence of the interaction.

After every interview, detailed field notes were made using a prepared 'field notes template'. This allowed a record to be made of such details as the researcher's reception (in the ward/home), the respondent's apparent mood and feelings, the interviewer's mood and feelings, any issues or difficulties that had emerged, comments offered and the quality of the tape recording. The unique character of each interview can be readily appreciated by consulting these field notes.

Before each audio-tape was transcribed in full directly into the computer analysis package, field notes from each interview were imported into the software where they were stored on the respondent's 'face card'. This approach allowed the researcher's account of each interaction, and the respondent's biographical and interview data, to be juxtaposed within the software. This reflected an effort to ensure that the analysis remained sensitive to the context within which the data were generated.

In the concluding stages of the interview, relatives commonly offered unsolicited reports that they had found the interview to be both comfortable and beneficial. After those interviews that were conducted in the homes, it was very common for the researcher to be engaged in social conversation with the respondent and during this time a number of relatives chose to show photographs of their dying relative.

The staff nurses

Acquiring the sample

Two staff nurses were recruited from each of eight study wards giving a total sample of 16 nurses. Staff nurses formed the sample because they were judged to be the group with the most direct patient and family contact and because, as mentors to students, they have considerable potential for influencing practice (Ceslowitz 1989). The decision to include two nurses from each ward was taken in an attempt to maintain continuity during the relatives' sample recruitment periods and the intervention. It was thus hoped that paired nurses could 'cover' for each other's days off, annual leave and night duty. Although it is possible that the potential success of the intervention might have been enhanced by involving all of the nurses from the eight ward teams, practical considerations relating to the very large numbers involved for interviewing, and the difficulties associated with releasing this number of staff to attend the workshop, precluded that option.

Subsequent to meeting with the researcher, the ward sisters/charge nurses discussed the study with their ward team and established which nurses might be interested in participating. The researcher was given names of two nurses from each ward and a personal introductory letter was sent to each of these nurses. Meetings were then arranged to allow the researcher to provide the staff nurses with further information about the study, to detail the level of involvement that would be required of the participating nurses and to seek their consent to be interviewed. On hearing what was involved, one nurse declined to participate and another from that ward volunteered to replace her. The others all agreed to participate and expressed interest in the study.

The staff nurses represented a diverse group in terms of age, sex, professional experience and educational background before and since entering nursing. The main characteristics of the staff nurses' sample are summarized in Table 4.3.

The staff nurses' interviews

The instruments

Two different staff nurse interview schedules were required: one for each phase of the study. The phase 1 instrument was developed around themes derived from the literature and used mainly open questions. The questions were designed to elicit (1) the nurses' feelings and concerns in relation to this aspect of their practice, (2) the nature and degree of stress that they experience when providing this form of care for the dying patient's family, and (3) the coping responses that they employ.

Although the themes summarized below were addressed in both phases of the study, the phase 2 interview schedule was shorter and focused mainly on the issues and concerns that had been raised in the nurses' phase 1 interviews. Questions were also included in the phase 2 instrument to allow exploration of the nurses' experiences of the workshop and acting in the role of facilitator during the intervention period of the study. In recognition of the potential for the extended relationship between the researcher and the staff nurses to influence the nurses' responses, questions were specifically worded to facilitate both positive and negative responses.

Themes addressed in the staff nurses' interviews
- Terminal care in the ward
- Relatives around the ward
- Facilities for families

Table 4.3: Sample profile of the staff nurses

Age range (years)		Staff nurse grade		Sex distribution	
21–26	6	D	3	Female	16
27–32	11	E	15	Male	2
33–38	0				
≥39	1				

Post-school qualifications on entry to RGN training		Years since registration	
		1–4	12
MA in History	1	5–8	4
Bachelor of Arts	1	> 8	2
Higher Nat. Dip. in Biology	1		
Enrolled Nurse	2	*Years in present post*	
Registered Mental Health Nurse	2	1–3 years	12
Registered Sick Children's Nurse	1	4–7 years	6

Post-registration studies

Studies undertaken/underway at the start of the current study	Number of nurses
Master's Degree studies	1
Registered Midwife (RM)	3

NBS Diploma in Professional Studies

One or more modules undertaken	10
None	8

Short courses and study days

Mentorship course	7
Project 2000 preparation	4
Lifting and handling course	5
Standard setting	3
Introduction to palliative care	1
Oncology/chemotherapy	1
Terminal care	1

Studies undertaken during the course of the current study

Standard setting study day	3
4-day oncology course	1
Terminal care study day	1
Palliative care conference	3
Professional studies (medical nursing)	1

- Staff–relative interface
- Information channels
- Nurses' experience of stress
- Coping responses
- Education and training
- Interprofessional issues.

The interview approach

The nurses' interviews were all conducted within the ward area. Although interview dates and times were negotiated in advance to ensure the least possible disruption to the ward routine, difficulties were at times encountered in relation to having to relieve the nurses of their duties for the interviews. Three nurses opted to be interviewed once their span of duty had been completed. Also, in some wards, finding a private area to conduct the interviews proved problematic and interruptions occurred during several interviews.

The nurses' interviews were audio-taped and transcribed in full into the computer analysis package. The interview schedule, although apparently very structured in design, was used as a framework and the nurses' interviews were conducted using an informal style that facilitated a steady flow of dialogue. The procedure for transcribing the audio-tapes, and for recording the interview field notes, followed the same pattern as that described above for the relatives.

Ethical considerations

A number of ethical issues needed to be addressed in relation to this study. Relatives who agreed to participate in the current study were judged likely to be vulnerable as a result of the stress associated with their current situation and their impending loss. The staff nurses were also judged to be vulnerable as a result of their exacting role in the study, which included participating in two interviews, approaching relatives to offer letters from the researcher and acting as facilitators/change agents in their wards during the intervention period.

As the study required the participation of vulnerable subjects, applications were lodged with both hospitals ethics committees and ethical approval was granted.

The National Commission for the Protection of Human Subjects of Biomedical and Behavioural Research identified a number of key ethical principles which should underpin the conduct of research with human subjects (Beauchamp and Childness 1983; Burns and Grove 1993). These principles are explored briefly below.

'Respect for Persons' represents the guiding ethical principle in relation to research with humans (Downie and Telfer 1980). 'Respect for Persons' holds that research participants have certain rights which must not be infringed either by the researcher or by the research process. These rights include rights to autonomy – to be self-determining and self-governing – rights to beneficence and non-maleficence, and that the researcher should be motivated to do good and above all to do no harm. Finally, research participants have a right to justice, i.e. to be treated at all times with fairness (Burns and Grove 1993, pp. 94–5). The key principles outlined above are considered in relation to the current study.

Respect for Persons

Within the framework of this over-arching ethical principle, issues will be considered in relation to research participants' autonomy, beneficence (and non-maleficence), and justice.

Autonomy

Informed consent : The notion of informed consent is central to autonomy and self-determination. Guidelines were followed to ensure that adequate information was provided to enable participants to give truly informed consent (Burns and Grove 1993). Participants received written and verbal information about the aims of the study, the criteria for selecting study participants and details of what would be required of participants. A consent form, designed using guidelines provided by the ethics committee, was signed by all participants. Before signing the consent form all participants were given the opportunity to meet with the researcher, so that clarification could be offered and questions answered.

Confidentiality: The promise of confidentiality was emphasized in bold type in the introductory letter and on the consent form. This was repeated verbally during the initial contact with the researcher and again at the start of the interview. Participants' identities were concealed using coded identification.

Beneficence and justice

Benefits of the study: It is an ethical imperative that participation in a research study should yield more good than harm for the individuals involved (Archbold 1986; Aranda, 1995). The current study goes beyond merely describing people's experiences and problems, and aims to discover ways to improve practice in the area of family support during terminal illness. Accordingly, the relatives were informed that, although they might not benefit personally from their participation in the study, it was hoped that care for relatives of very ill patients might in the future improve as a result of the study. It is also reported in Chapter 6 that ethical concerns relating to benefi-cence arose during the intervention, which caused the evaluation research approach to be altered so that the study could be conducted within an action research framework.

Coercion: When recruiting relatives for the study, it was judged important that they should be able to decline without discomfort. To this end the introductory letter emphasized in bold type that relatives must not feel under any pressure to participate and must indeed feel free to decline. The nurses were also fully briefed, both verbally and in writing, about the approach that they should adopt when offering relatives a letter. The nurses' role was to deliver the letter in a sensitive manner, at a time when the relative was away from the bedside and preferably just before he or she left the ward. It was emphasized that it was *not* the nurses' role to urge relatives to participate in the study. A return slip allowed those relatives who agreed to a preliminary contact to select whether this should be by the researcher telephoning them or by her meeting them at the ward entrance at an agreed date and time. Only after this initial contact was established were relatives asked if they would be willing to participate in the study.

Exploitation: Interviewing vulnerable people raises a number of complex ethical issues. A dilemma exists between, on the one hand, facilitating the expression of the interviewee's experiences and feel-ings and, on the other, provoking catharsis, perhaps causing hard-won emotional control to be lost. Also, decisions had to be taken about how to respond should a participant become upset during an interview. During the pilot study the researcher's response to signs of distress was to redirect the questions. As a result of these avoidance tactics, the quality of the interaction and the data were at times adversely affected.

This tension was resolved by encouraging respondents to take control of the pace and depth of the interaction. At the start of each interview the respondent was informed that he or she must feel absolutely free to decline to answer any question, or to stop the interview at any time, should he or she wish to do so. At several points during the interview, respondents were asked 'Is it all right for us to go on?' or 'Would you prefer that we stop now?'. In the event none of the participants terminated the interview or declined to answer any question, and with experience the interviewer accepted and offered support during natural expressions of sadness.

A study of this nature carries a significant risk that vulnerable participants might be exploited. The following measures were taken in an effort to counter this risk. Within 24 hours of the interview, a hand-written notelet was sent to the relative to express the researcher's appreciation. The researcher's work address and telephone number were included on the note and several people did use these to initiate further contact. After the death of the patient, a simple letter of condolence was also sent. In these small ways it was hoped to convey sensitivity and to acknowledge the relatives' valued contribution to the study.

After the interview, in situations where it was judged to be appropriate, relatives were asked if they would be willing to participate in a second short interview in 2 weeks time if their loved one was still in the ward at that time. All of the relatives very readily agreed to this.

Rationale for the second interview

A second interview was suggested for two reasons: the first methodological and the second ethical. It was judged that the dynamic nature of the relatives' situation might mean that their experiences and feelings could change over time, especially as the death of their loved one drew nearer. The second reason for offering a second interview was ethical and was intended to avoid the situation where, after a lengthy and often emotionally charged encounter, the researcher abruptly severed contact with the respondent. The second interviews differed in character from the first, tending more towards the counselling rather than the research interview mode. This change in focus was largely initiated by the relatives who all reported that they welcomed the opportunity to re-establish contact. The data clearly reveal that the relatives used their second interview as an opportunity to seek support.

Analysis processes

The analysis techniques described below were applied during both phases of the study and with both the nurses' and the relatives' interview data.

The selection and operational characteristics of the analysis software have already been described when reporting the pilot study (see p. 65) and are not repeated here. The following section focuses more specifically on how the data were handled during the analysis and interpretative processes undertaken during the main study.

Every interview was transcribed in full directly into Hyperqual2.1, a computer textual analysis package (Padilla 1993), together with the accompanying field notes, thus generating a considerable volume of data. Verbal utterances and audible emotional expressions such as laughing, weeping or sighing were also recorded, and silences and pauses were represented by dots to indicate the length of the pause. In each phase of the study, two 'parent' stacks were created to receive the data: one for nurses, the other for relatives. Copies were then made of the two newly created stacks and the originals were locked to prevent their being changed or erased. Thereafter analysis was conducted on the duplicate stacks.

A total of 80 interviews were audio-taped, transcribed and analysed: 44 in phase 1 of the study and 36 in phase 2. Each interview represented a unique, personal contribution and only after responding to and interpreting each transcript in its own right were comparisons made across the data set(s).

Analysis was conducted in a series of stages during which the transcripts were repeatedly and intensively scrutinized. Transcripts were first read through in full and typing errors were corrected. The next stage represented a 'global analysis', during which the transcripts were examined scrupulously line by line as the audio-tapes were simultaneously played to confirm the context. At this early stage, emerging ideas and impressions were recorded alongside the text in the 'notes field'. The analysis program offered the facility of a question-by-question printout of all of the respondents' answers to each individual question, together with the analyst's comments, which had been recorded in the notes field. This facility was particularly useful with questions that had yielded copious data. Using these hard copies, similarities and differences between respondents could be demonstrated and possible links to biographical or other factors explored. Also, by providing an unabridged version of the responses, the context was retained.

As analysis progressed, significant segments of text were highlighted and 'tagged'. Using these tags as 'search strings', the stack could be searched and segments of similar data located, copied and exported to form new homogeneous 'exemplar stacks'. Exemplar stacks formed the cornerstone of analysis. As the analysis became increasingly focused, new stacks were formed and new perceptions gained. Metaphors in the respondents' language often yielded startling insights into the feelings of the participants.

Thematically related exemplars were printed and this proved to be a very powerful tool in the interpretative process. Stacks could also be merged to link similar data or to collapse related themes. The analyst could navigate with ease both within and between stacks and this ability to maintain links between segments of text and the main stack meant that contextual links could be preserved.

Analysis of the relatives' and nurses' phase 1 data was an emotionally and intellectually intensive activity which yielded powerful data. In the quest for deeper understanding of the emerging issues and themes, the researcher repeatedly returned to the literature. During the course of the phase 1 analysis, it was becoming increasingly evident to the researcher that the analysis approach was changing and evolving in response to the compelling data that were emerging. Acknowledgement of these perceptual shifts led the researcher to further study of the methods literature.

Subsequent reflections on insights gained from the literature confirmed that the analysis processes currently being employed showed strong parallels with the hermeneutic approach to interpretative analysis. Although the original study plan did not incorporate a phenomenological design, examination of the tapes and transcripts revealed that the question form used, and the interview approach adopted, resulted in substantial access into the experiences and feelings of both the relatives and the nurses. These unanticipated developments, which represented a reflexive response to the powerful phase 1 data, offered insights into the phenomenological method. Literature consulted in the course of reaching this new awareness is reported in the next section.

Hermeneutic phenomenology

The term 'hermeneutics' can be traced to Greek mythology where Hermes, a messenger associated with the Delphic Oracle, was responsible for changing the 'unknowable' into a form that humans could understand (Wilson and Hutchieson 1991). Leonard (1989), retaining this original essence, defines hermeneutics as 'interpretation of language so that that which was foreign to our experience is made comprehensible'. Hermeneutic phenomenology represents a departure from 'pure' phenomenology in terms of the researcher's relationship to, and knowledge of, the phenomena under investigation. Husserl's position was that the researcher should adopt a 'presuppositionless' stance and set aside or 'bracket' prior knowledge, attitudes or experience, so that the phenomenon is approached in an open manner (Schutz 1970; Reeder 1987). The Heideggerian view challenges this position, accepting that the investigator's professional background, life experience and prior knowledge of the subject must inevitably be brought to the phenomenon under study (Wrubel et al. 1981; Atwood and Hinds 1986; Benner 1994).

Phenomenology and nursing

Thorne (1991) argues that, as it is nursing's obligation and privilege to be a practical rather than a purely theoretical enterprise, our professional biases demand that nursing research has practical applicability. This demand for utility has a bearing on the types of phenomenological enquiry that nurses require or will accept (Thorne 1991). Rather than seeking to understand the deeper structures of 'being', nurse phenomenologists have tended to use the approach to explore and illuminate subjective experiences within everyday nursing practice (Swanson-Kauffman and Schonwald 1988; Walters 1994; Wros 1994).

The hermeneutic research interview

The hermeneutic interview is characterized by a methodological consciousness which is clearly reflected in the question form, and in the researcher's critical awareness of the complex interactions that operate within every research encounter (Kvale 1983). The central purpose of the hermeneutic interview is to achieve understanding about the interviewee's life world. In contrast with questionnaire or content analysis approaches, the approach should be truly qualitative. Interviews are usually semi-structured and typically last from 1 to 2 hours. In some cases, if the respondent so chooses or is especially self-reflective, repeat interviews may be useful (Wilson and Hutchieson 1991). Questions should focus on specific themes and the interviewer should guide the conversation around these themes, but should not guide the interviewee's opinions of the themes (Kvale 1983). The resulting transcripts, audio-tapes and field notes all represent data for interpretation. The emerging data should be theme oriented, contextual and accurately reflect the interviewee's subjective experience (Kvale 1983). In contrast with the pre-suppositionless stance of 'pure' phenomenology, a degree of reflexivity is seen as a strength in the hermeneutic approach. Indeed, Kvale (1983) suggests that a well-carried-through interview could be a positive experience for the respondent because, for most people, to have the undivided attention of another who is willing to listen with interest for between 1 and 2 hours can be a rare and enriching experience.

Interpretative analysis

Hermeneutic principles imply a particular approach to the interpretation of text (Kvale 1983). The interpreter approaches the data with 'wide-open eyes' and engages in a process of intense reflection. Interpretation requires insight, imagination, openness and patience in order to acquire the art of understanding (Reeder 1988). Analysis is intensely demanding of energy and time, and is usually terminated by time limit or exhaustion rather than by a sense that the fullest possible understanding has been reached. The analyst's understanding of the respondent's world is deepened through interpretation of emerging themes, and this interpretation is taken to an even deeper level and further illumination is sought by drawing on relevant theory (Kvale 1983). Textual analysis is a dynamic process in which the researcher enters the 'hermeneutic circle' where the analyst constantly moves between segments of text and the whole text, thus allowing interpretations to be viewed in their fullest context. In interpretative analysis the researcher becomes co-creator of the text and his or her pre-suppositions are fully accepted (Kvale 1983; Reeder 1988; Leonard 1994; Walters 1994).

Hermeneutic interpretation begins with an initial global analysis, which involves a slow careful scrutiny of the whole text (Leonard 1994). At this point the interpreter will be 'hyper-attending' and new perspectives, insights and understandings are gained from the emerging themes. Interpretation of these themes leads the researcher to identify specific exemplars and paradigm cases. These represent strong instances that capture the meaning of a situation in a way that it is instantly recognizable to the reader and yet does not distort or decontextualize the experience. Presentation of the findings requires distillation of the data to their most essential terms, while leaving enough evidence for validation processes to be undertaken (Leonard 1994).

Reinharz (1983) encapsulates the key principles of the hermeneutic approach by describing it as a series of 'transformations'.

The hermeneutic approach as transformation

- The respondent transforms his or her feelings and experiences into language
- The researcher interprets the conversation or text
- The researcher's interpretations are transformed into themes that provide insights
- The themes are transformed into a meaningful account that enables new knowledge and understanding to be communicated
- The final transformation occurs when the reader or listener creates their own interpretations and acts on them (Reinharz 1983).

Rigour and truth worthiness

Science is not a set of techniques but is rather a state of mind

(Mays and Pope 1995, p. 109)

As the primary aim of qualitative research is to study people within their unique context, the notion of a subjective, multi-perspective view of a phenomenon is fully accepted (Kvale 1983; Baker et al. 1992). As naturalistic enquiry rests on completely different assumptions from those of the opposite (positivist) paradigm, there seems to be no logical reason to apply identical validity and reliability rules and criteria. Sandelowski (1986) asserts that applying the criteria of one research tradition to another merely amounts to self-justification. Rigour in qualitative methods should therefore be evaluated using methodologically appropriate criteria such as those of credibility, truth worthiness, applicability and auditability (Sandelowski 1986; Guba and Lincoln 1994). Credibility and truth worthiness are enhanced when the investigator clearly explicates the methodological approach and the theoretical underpinnings of the study, and when the findings are presented in an honest way (Leininger 1984). Rigour is also enhanced when the researcher maintains meticulous records that offer a clear, auditable account of contextual issues and the research strategies and that clearly describe the analysis techniques. To this end all audio-tapes, field notes and transcripts should be made available for scrutiny by an auditor (Altheide and Johnson 1994).

In the current study, 44 of the audio-tapes were transcribed by the researcher and the remaining 36 by a typist. The researcher's judgement is that the quality of analysis was not significantly affected by having personally transcribed the tapes. However, an issue that did arise was the effect of the subject matter on the transcriber. One typist had to stop the work as she found the relatives' accounts too distressing.

An experienced qualitative researcher agreed to undertake an audit of the research processes and to judge the truth worthiness and credibility of the findings. This person was invited to select audio-tapes, transcripts and field notes to confirm that the transcription accurately represented the interaction, that the analysis approach and techniques were appropriate and rigorous, and that the researcher's interpretations were credible.

Furthermore, each exemplar used to support the account has been labelled with its precise source in terms of the interview number, question number and card number from which the quote was extracted. The strategy of labelling exemplars in this way was adopted primarily to retain the link between each exemplar and the full account, thus retaining the context from which it was drawn, but it was also hoped that this labelling process would enable the reader to see the range of sources from which similar data had been drawn and to permit areas of commonality and uniqueness to be revealed.

By using the electronic linkages provided by the software, and also by closely scrutinizing hard copies of thematically related data, pre- and post-intervention experiences and views could be interpreted from the dual perspectives of the nurses and relatives, e.g. if a nurse in a given ward claimed that positive changes had occurred in the ward in relation to communications with relatives, then relatives' reported experiences in that ward could be consulted to seek corroboration of the claim for positive change. This approach, which follows the conventions of hermeneutic analysis, involved a constant moving forward and back between the whole and the parts of each individual account, between pre- and post-intervention data, and between nurses' and relatives' data. These complex interpretative processes were greatly facilitated by the computerized form of analysis that was adopted in the study.

A colleague, who is an experienced nurse researcher and committed phenomenologist, and whose own PhD studies and subsequent writings are based on Heideggerian hermeneutics, regularly permitted the researcher to subject her reasoning and emerging understanding to his scrutiny and counsel.

Another colleague from the psychology department, whose own PhD study employed stress and coping as the theoretical framework, agreed to act as an adviser. Her advice was particularly valuable in relation to the interpretative analysis where links with the theoretical framework of stress and coping were being explored.

The role of theory in qualitative work

Controversy exists about how central theory ought to be within the structure of a research project and whether methodological rigour is enhanced by firm theoretical adherence. Sandelowski (1993a) argues that, in qualitative research, theory can be employed on a number of different levels where it may be used either centrally or peripherally within a research project – she describes the more peripheral use of theory as 'brush stroking the theory in to enhance interpretation'. Kvale (1983) further suggests that hermeneutic interpretation is enlarged and enriched by drawing on wider knowledge which is often an amalgam of the researcher's experience and extant theory. A number of nursing scholars have sought deeper understanding of a range of phenomena by applying a blend of theories such as stress and coping or human caring theory, with philosophies such as phenomenology, and the understanding that has been gained from their scholarship has been widely applied within the service of nursing (Wrubel et al. 1981; Watson 1988; Benner and Wrubel 1989; Clarke and Wheeler 1992; Darbyshire 1992; Wros 1993; Walters 1994).

The theoretical and philosophical underpinnings applied within the current study, and in particular the interpretative approach employed when analysing the nurses' and relatives' data, closely follow the central tenets of the cognitive phenomenological transactional theories of stress and coping explicated by Wrubel et al. (1981). This theoretical and philosophical approach, fully described in Chapter 3, permits stressful experiences to be interpreted within their fullest possible context. It furthermore acknowledges the reciprocal and reflexive nature of the relationships that operate within every stressful encounter, and recognizes that each situation will be appraised from the unique and subjective perspective of the person involved.

Authenticity and applicability

Reeder (1988) believes that skilful use of language in a research report can have the power to impassion, empower and awaken the sensitivity of the reader to the human condition. Exemplars and paradigm cases offer a vivid means of extending understanding so that it may be converted into meaningful action within nursing practice (Benner 1983; Wros 1993). Guba and Lincoln (1994) describe the researcher's role in reporting this kind of work as that of a passionate participant who actively facilitates the multi-voice. They argue that, when readers respond to the research account, reconstructions are formed, change is facilitated and individuals are stimulated to take action (Guba and Lincoln 1994). A research report that can move the reader to action is said to have 'catalytic authenticity', whereas the term 'tactical authenticity' describes the capacity of research findings to empower action (Guba and Lincoln 1994). Kvale (1983) describes six different levels of hermeneutic interpretation and he claims that the deepest level occurs when participants respond to research data by extending their own interpretations into corrective action in the form of action research.

In Chapter 6, it is reported that it was precisely this type of empowerment, generated by their response to the phase 1 interview data that resulted in the staff nurses extending their interpretations of the data into dynamic and collaborative action aimed at changing the nature of their practice and the quality of their care.

Chapter 5
Phase 1 findings

The relatives' accounts

As stated in Chapter 4, a total of 26 relatives' interviews were conducted during phase 1 of the study. The interview schedule incorporates a number of key themes and concepts of interest which also provide the framework through which the main theoretical aspects of the study are explored. This chapter reports the findings from the relatives' phase 1 interviews and incorporates a number of major themes, each of which is described in turn. These include the relatives' experiences before admission, the way the hospital admission was perceived, the relatives' experiences of facilities and communications, and their coping strategies and support needs. The major themes and subthemes to emerge from the analysis of the relatives' phase 1 interviews are summarized in Table 5.1.

Table 5.1: Themes and subthemes in the relatives' accounts

Preadmission experience	Impact of the diagnosis
	The cancer journey
	The burden of care
Hospital as sanctuary	Crisis intervention
	Feelings in conflict
	Facilities and care
Staff–relative interface	Initiating contact
	Communication/information
	Smooth paths or brick walls?
Relatives' stress	Emotional impact
	Physical health
	Socioeconomic impact
Coping and support	Strategies for coping
	Access to support
	Needs – met and unmet

Thematic analysis

The preadmission experience

The relatives, without exception, sought to place their current experiences in context by referring back, often at some length, to their experiences during the early stages in the patients' illnesses. Although for some the unexpected diagnosis had come as a shock, for others the news merely confirmed their suspicions. The data offered revealing insights into the effects that receiving such news had on the relatives. This is illustrated below as a woman describes receiving her husband's grave prognosis. She had received this information only 8 weeks before the interview.

> It was Christmas Eve when the doctor told me they had drained his lung and they felt sure that he had cancer. I said 'No . . . *No* . . . *that's not true*' On Boxing Day I had another word with the doctor and he told me that Jack had only a few weeks to live. He said 'if you have any family abroad you should get in touch'.
>
> Interview no. 1

Although the relatives had all experienced a degree of shock when informed of the diagnosis, they then entered a period of adjustment to the illness. However, this adaptation was not straightforward because, as the patient passed through various stages of the disease, with symptoms being at times quiescent and at others more intrusive, the relatives' emotional responses alternated between hope and despair. In the following exemplars the relatives describe precisely that kind of experience.

> Well, he had his first operation 5 years ago. Then in May he was brought back in again, and he got a double dosage of radium and he was let home again. Since then it's just been a matter of attending to him. For four years now I've been running . . . .
>
> Interview no. 16

> This is the fourth or fifth time I have been told that my husband has about 10 days or 24 hours (to live). Really . . . there's a saturation point that you get to. It's bad enough . . . it really is a shock the first time, let me tell you. But to be told this about 3 or 4 times is really a bit much. There's a limit to what you can cope with.
>
> Interview no. 10

The data offered evidence of the difficulties that relatives face while caring for their loved one at home. As the patients' conditions worsened and their problems intensified, the degree of distress and the physical and mental exhaustion that many care-giving relatives experienced is described by a 70-year-old who had cared for her husband until the week before he died.

> He started complaining of pains in his stomach but he couldn't get to the toilet and he messed himself . . . and he was crying. I told him not to worry and got him in the bath He was in the bath and was rubbing my face saying 'This shouldn't be happening. You shouldn't have to do this for me.' That happened a lot that Sunday [diarrhoea and incontinence] and I couldn't get through to my doctor – I kept ringing, and ringing and ringing . . . I thought – this is *terrible*.
>
> Interview no. 2

Hospital as sanctuary

With only one exception hospital admission had represented crisis intervention. Relatives reported increasing difficulties as the patients' conditions worsened, symptoms became more difficult to control and care demands escalated. In the exemplar below, the 'relative' was in fact a life-long friend who, despite living some distance from the patient, had accepted responsibility for his care.

> He was admitted after us being there [in casualty] for about 4 hours. I was very relieved. Very, very relieved. By that time we were just desperate for somebody to do something to help him.
>
> Interview no. 7

The stress that relatives experienced when they could no longer adequately relieve the patient's distress was clearly evident. Severe pain, vomiting and breathing difficulties represented the most common examples of symptoms that the caring relatives could not bring under control. Situations similar to the one described below were reported by around two-thirds of the sample.

> He did have pain and he was really very very short of breath. The GP was going to leave him for 48 hours but he decided that he would need to come right in. His breathing was really very, very bad.
>
> Interview no. 2

One woman, who had been very anxious to continue to provide care for her mother, expressed strong feelings of frustration when her plans to 'care to the end' had to be abandoned. In the exemplar below, she describes the traumatic events that led to her mother's urgent, and final, admission to hospital.

> She started coughing and then the thing burst [possibly an abscess associated with the tumour]. And the *stench* . . . . We got the GP and she said 'she would be better in hospital 'til they clear this infection'. I was vomiting with the stench it was so . . . horrendous. [voice shaking]
>
> Interview no. 20

Feelings in conflict

The complex and conflicting array of feelings that the hospital admission had generated was clearly revealed in the data. As they came to acknowledge that they could no longer, with confidence, ensure the comfort and safety of their loved ones, the relatives commonly reported experiencing conflicting emotions. The three exemplars below are strongly representative of the types of responses reported by the relatives.

> I feel in a way relieved that she's in here and yet in a way I feel guilty too. Because I was the one that was always there. I still miss her . . . [struggling for control] You know? . . . but I feel as if some of the worry has been taken off me. It was all getting a wee bit too much for me.
>
> Interview no. 3

> I have to admit I feel guilty. He's gone downhill so fast that I can't help wondering if the strain of bringing him in has speeded things up . . . And yet I know full well that's not true . . . I *know* it's not. And I know I brought him in for his benefit. I know I don't have anything to feel guilty about. But I still feel it. Though I know in my heart that I have nothing to feel guilty about it's still there.
>
> Interview no. 23

The following exemplar offers revealing insight into the relative's emotional reactions in the lead-up to her loved one's death.

> I walk down the road and see dirty old men sitting with wine bottles and I think . . . I mean I *know* I shouldn't be like that but I say to myself 'you're sitting there like that and my husband is dying in hospital'. And then I go to chapel and I ask God to forgive me.
>
> Interview no. 2

The extent of the distress conveyed by these data provide reminders, confirmed in the literature, that, in the period leading up to the death of a loved one, close family members experience profound emotions such as feelings of anger and injustice associated with grief reactions (Hackett and Weisman 1985; Morris 1988; Simpson 1989). The data have confirmed that relatives of patients dying in hospital commonly experience significant distress. It was therefore judged important to elicit the relatives' views about the support and facilities that the hospitals provided, especially when extended periods of time were spent in the wards in the days leading up to the death of their loved one.

Facilities for families

With the worsening of their loved one's condition, many relatives spent increasing lengths of time in the wards. All but one of the relatives interviewed were in this category and just under half had stayed overnight in the ward. Both positive and negative comments were received about the facilities that were provided for them at this time. The most frequent comments received related to their difficulties in obtaining access to refreshments and to a private area for discussions with staff. Relatives who stayed overnight also commented on their problems gaining access to a private area where they could withdraw from the bedside for periods of rest and to manage their distress. There was, however, evidence in these data that, in many wards, the nurses made considerable efforts to keep relatives supplied with light refreshments and that this was much appreciated. The comment below is representative of several others.

> I must admit the staff were very good because they did pop in and offer us tea and coffee at any time. They even offered us food.
>
> Interview no. 10

Negative comments about the provision of facilities were, however, received by almost half the respondents. The exemplars below, both from elderly relatives, highlight the main issues of concern.

> Facilities for relatives are nil. Absolutely nil. To get a cup of tea or go to the toilet you've to go away down to the ground floor. There's nothing at all on the ward level. Things are sadly lacking in that sense. There's no facilities at all for people.
>
> Interview no. 21

If you just had a wee sort of room. You know? Even just a wee camp bed or
something that you could lie out on . . . just to stretch out. That's the main problem. Because you're all hunched up all night, and your back, your hips and your
thighs get all stiff.

Interview no. 18

In the exemplar below, a woman describes her experiences
when she stayed for several days and nights at the bedside of her
dying mother. Although this represents a single incident, it has
been included because it offers a graphic illustration of unmet
need for sensitive and supportive care for the dying patient's
family.

I asked for a pillow and the nurse said 'I'll see if I can get one for you'. When she
came back she said, 'I had to get that pillow from another ward. I had to sign for
it and I've to take it back first thing in the morning.' At 7 o'clock she was back
and took my pillow away from me. I thought that was terrible . . . . I used to sit
at night without pillows. I sat up in the chair all night.

Interview no. 20

Unmet needs for support from medical staff were also reported.
In the example below an elderly woman reports her reactions to a
conversation that took place in the corridor between herself and
the senior consultant who was looking after her husband. During
that communication she was informed of her husband's grave
prognosis.

There was nowhere where you could go to be alone for a minute or two. I mean
what would that doctor have done if I had fallen at his feet or burst into floods of
tears? I just flew for my daughter and we had a cup of tea in the staff canteen . .
. . But even there you had no privacy. I mean she was crying and I was crying
and you'd nowhere you could go.

Interview no. 21

Although the relatives' judgements about facilities were overwhelmingly negative, several were at pains to express the view that
the nurses were not to blame for the poor provision of facilities in
hospital. However, the fact that over a third of the relatives reported
difficulties in gaining access to a private area raises a number of
important issues that have a bearing on communication.

Establishing contact with staff

The data confirm the findings in the literature (Northouse and Northouse 1987; Lugton 1989a) that relatives commonly experience difficulties in knowing just how to initiate contact with staff. The relatives, almost unanimously, described feeling hesitant about 'making the first move'. It was very common indeed for relatives to express concerns about disturbing 'busy nurses' whom they perceived to be involved in activities too important to be interrupted. Although there was evidence that relatives did feel the need for regular face-to-face contact with nursing staff, more than two-thirds of the sample expressed concern that they might be seen as a nuisance if they approached the staff too frequently. Some of these concerns are illustrated in the exemplars below.

> It's knowing just who it is you should approach. Because now you have so many sisters, staff nurses and what have you, you cannot identify one person as the person that you should speak to. And I don't like approaching them [nurses] in case they're too busy with something else. So I appreciate it when they say to me 'Excuse me, could I have a word with you?' Yes I appreciate that.
>
> Interview no. 17

> If families were told at the outset that the nurses were there, that they could be approached with any questions, any worries, if they knew that from the outset and were reminded of it from time to time. Especially if you didn't come forward and ask anything.
>
> Interview no. 7

When asked how they actually 'went about' getting to speak to staff, some relatives explained how they came to their decisions about whom they should approach. They revealed how they watched the staff closely to pick up cues from their manner, to help them to judge who might be most approachable, e.g. although nurses with an open and friendly style conveyed a sense of accessibility, those who rarely made eye contact or smiled caused relatives to feel hesitant about approaching them. The relative speaking below illustrates this very clearly.

> There are some nurses that you would approach more readily than others. It really depends on their attitude. If you feel that their attitude is good and that

they're quite happy to talk to you, then that's the one you'll seek out. The attitude of the nursing staff is really important.

Interview no. 4

Access to information

Relatives overwhelmingly stated the need for regular information about their loved one's care and progress, and it was clear from their comments that they would prefer information to be offered rather than having to seek it out. The need for some continuity of information was also expressed, with around half of the sample suggesting that they would appreciate regular contact with the same member of staff. Relatives' needs in this regard are illustrated in the following quotes.

Maybe if they had a certain person appointed for each shift to liaise with the family and to give them . . . to voluntarily give them information.

Interview no. 3

There is one staff nurse who's just like an oasis. She seeks me out and gives me little bits of information so I know what's going on.

Interview no. 1

They're very good. The staff nurse especially. She's been really good. My sister and I think she's marvellous. She explains everything to us. I mean she doesn't just say we've given her methadone, she tells us what it's doing for her.

Interview no. 11

The data revealed that relatives' information needs were complex. Although, on some days, relatives reported the need for very detailed information, at other times they only wanted a basic report about the patient's comfort. The comment offered below underlines the relatives' fluctuating capacity to confront the reality of their situation. This raises the question about whether relatives might benefit from being given greater control over the processes of information exchange.

Sometimes you don't want to hear. I suppose it's just that there are some days when you feel that you can't take too much detail.

Interview no. 3

The above exemplar serves as a reminder that the sustained stress imposed by terminal illness on a loved one can take its toll on the relatives' emotional and physical health and well-being. In the current study, this was compounded by the fact, confirmed in the phase 1 relatives' sample profile, that over half of the relatives of dying patients are themselves elderly.

Impact on health and well-being

At the time of their interview, several relatives were receiving medical treatment for a variety of ongoing medical disorders. Reported conditions included diabetes mellitus, duodenal ulcer, cervical spondylitis and a cardiac arrhythmia being treated with a pacemaker. The sample also included an elderly man only partially recovered from a recent stroke.

Without exception the relatives reported feeling 'exhausted', 'worn out' or 'drained'. All reported sleeping little and badly, and most were not eating normally. Concentration and memory were generally described as very poor and several relatives reported feeling irritable and depressed. The exemplars below highlight the sort of problems that were reported

> I have angina and recently I have had to take more tablets and sleep propped up. I feel drained at times. Really drained. I find that I have to rest in the mornings. You just have to pace yourself.
>
> Interview no. 9

> I'm not taking my medicine as I should do because I forget. I've got so many other things on my mind. I have to take this tablet in the morning to keep the blood pressure regular. I'm supposed to take it every day and I don't think I've had one for a week.
>
> Interview no. 21

> I am absolutely physically exhausted as well as emotionally. Last night I felt that I had come to a pitch where if I didn't put my head down I would fall down. Other nights my mind is so active that I find great difficulty in sleeping.
>
> Interview no. 2

The effects that stress can have on physical health has already been established in the literature (Selye 1974; Nixon 1993), and this is confirmed in the relatives' data. Two respondents vividly describe the physical manifestations of their stress.

> The doctor gave me tablets to relax me and calm me. Anti-anxiety pills they were. He said I was taking panic attacks. I thought I was taking a shock [lay term for a stroke]. All down one side was numb and I had pins and needles in my arms, and I felt as if my face was getting twisted on one side. The GP said it was nervous spasm that I was taking. I still take it if . . . if I think about things too much.
>
> Interview no. 1

> I've got syncope. Just passing out. I've had CAT scans and ECGs and everything's come back negative. I had a relapse the other night and collapsed in the toilet. I'm putting it all down to stress.
>
> Interview no. 20

Despite evidence of significant stress, family relationships were mainly reported as being closer and stronger than ever. However, in three families, conflicts had surfaced adding to the general distress, and in another family a relationship between father and daughter was being rebuilt during the father's terminal illness. The following quote offers a clear example of the support that can come from within the close family.

> The family have all been marvellous. My husband has been very supportive and my brother and sister have been forward and back from Canada quite a bit and of course we have all been in constant phone contact.
>
> Interview no. 3

A few relatives reported financial stress caused by the costs involved in travelling to and from the hospital and also as a result of loss of earnings. The sample contained several families who would have appreciated a referral to the Hospital Social Worker for help and advice about financial difficulties. The relatives below offer examples of the potential economic consequences of terminal illness.

> I've been unemployed for some time and what with fares to the hospital and buying stuff to bring in . . . it fairly runs away with the money.
>
> Interview no. 17

> I had to give up my job and Jim had to give up his job too. He was planning to work on, because he was fit enough before it hit him. So that was two wages that we lost.
>
> Interview no. 18

In concurrence with theories reported in the literature, the data reveal the pervasive and transactional nature of the relatives' stress (Wrubel et al. 1981; Folkman 1984). Although their stress was primarily generated by their loved one's deteriorating health, and by their own impending loss, factors within the hospital environment and their own subjective responses to their situation were also influential. Some of the coping strategies that the relatives used to manage their stress are considered below.

Coping strategies

It has already been reported in the literature that individuals respond to stress using both problem-focused and emotion-focused coping strategies (Wrubel et al. 1981; Folkman, 1984). In the current study, the relatives' stress was primarily generated by the patient's impending death and, as this was a situation that relatives could not directly influence, problem-focused coping strategies were not very evident in their responses. There was, however, considerable evidence of emotion-focused strategies being used by every relative interviewed.

These strategies included seeking information, seeking support from family and others, and employing psychological defensive strategies such as avoidance. Several relatives reported that only by pushing the reality of their situation to the back of their mind could they manage to get through each day. The following woman offered a clear example of this coping strategy.

> I can go for days without getting upset and then maybe all of a sudden all I do is bubble [weep]. At times it's just not penetrating what's happening to her and then all of a sudden just the daftest wee thing brings it all back into focus.
>
> Interview no. 1

As death approached, several relatives reported a shift in coping behaviour. Rather than their previous strategies of keeping busy and seeking distraction, they became quieter and more reflective. At this stage all attempts at denial were finally shelved and the forthcoming death was acknowledged. The following two quotes illustrate this transition. In particular, the second woman describes mentally rehearsing for the next challenge ahead.

I used to find that if I was feeling under stress I'd start cleaning everything. Just keep busy . . . you know? But now if my mother . . . if she's worse . . . I can't do that any more . . . I want to do things yet I can't. I just want to sit and think about her.

Interview no. 13

My husband will say to me 'you're away in a dream'. God forgive me . . . I'm thinking about funerals. I mean she's still here and . . . I'm . . . I mean I can *see funerals*. Everything. I see all this in my mind.

Interview no. 4

Several relatives expressed the wish that it would soon be 'over' and, although a number of veiled references were made to euthanasia, the manner in which these were expressed revealed understandable ambivalence.

I met the doctor at the door and I said 'my mother is awful distressed I would rather you would give her something'. I meant give her something to put her away altogether [euthanasia]. I really did mean that at the time. But then when I saw her afterwards, after she'd calmed down, I was sorry I had said that.

Interview no. 1

Support needs

In concurrence with the reported literature (Hull 1989b), relatives in the current study reported that their greatest support came from seeing the patient being well cared for, with symptoms being adequately controlled. Although relatives consistently reported that their own needs were of lesser importance than the patient's, the current data reveal that relatives need to feel welcome in the ward, to have free access to their loved one and to receive regular, and up-to-date, information about the patient. Relatives also appreciated and gained support from staff who took time to talk to them and listen to their concerns. Two relatives would have appreciated information about a support group and two others would have welcomed advice about what to do following the patient's death. The need for this type of support is vividly described by a man whose wife was very close to death.

If there was just somebody that you could go to . . . [control very fragile] to give you advice about funeral arrangements . . . Because I've not got a clue . . . I'll sort it out right enough . . . but just at the moment . . . . Maybe it would help in this situation to get even a booklet that you could read at home.

Interview no. 17

Final comments

As each interview was brought to a close, the respondent was asked if there was anything that he or she wanted to add to what had been said. This final part of the interview sometimes contained quite lengthy comments, with the relative often spontaneously sharing information about their loved one's personal qualities and about their relationship with the patient. Most commonly, the relatives offered personal and sometimes emotional appeals on behalf of their loved one and, less commonly, relatives offered pleas on their own behalf. Relatives seemed to need reassurance that, if they had to leave the patient for any reason, there would be someone in the ward who would truly care *about* and for their loved one until they returned. The following two respondents illustrate this need.

> He needs someone to hug him and more time spent with him. And these girls are so hard worked. They don't have the time to spend with him
>
> Interview no. 16

> I would ask them to try to look beyond the difficulties that they're experiencing with this particular person and see that, well if there are relatives and friends who care so much for him, there must be more to them than they're seeing at this point of time. Some of them do know that . . . . And although I'm talking of my particular old man now, and although he has not always been an easy old man to deal with, we all love him dearly. He is a very loveable old man.
>
> Interview no. 14

Many appreciative comments, such as the example below, were made during this closing stage of the interview.

> I'm totally satisfied with them. They've been excellent, from doctors down to the wee woman who sweeps the floor. Everyone has been exceptionally good.
>
> Interview no. 18

Although criticisms were few, and tended to be offered hesitantly, those that were received underlined the extent of the distress that relatives of dying patients can experience. The quote below offers a particularly strong example.

> There are a lot of changes needed. Definitely. When I was in that room with my mother I was alone. It was just her and me. I was alone. Very, very much alone.
>
> Interview no. 20

Conclusion

When reporting the findings of the relatives' phase 1 analysis, a representative sample of the views and feelings expressed has been offered. The data seem to confirm that the dying patient's relatives commonly experience personal and family distress which goes right back to the time of their loved one's diagnosis. Consequently relatives of dying patients often enter the hospital system already vulnerable and are frequently experiencing conflicting and distressing emotions.

These data confirm that establishing contact with staff, and gaining access to regular information, is not straightforward. Difficulties in gaining access to facilities for the family's basic comfort and privacy were also highlighted. In addition, the relatives without exception reported significant stress that was found to have physical, psychological and socioeconomic dimensions. Although the nature of their situation placed considerable limitations on the coping options that were available to them, the data revealed that, under current care provision, a proportion of the relatives' needs remained unmet.

The staff nurses' accounts

As stated in Chapter 4, 18 staff nurses' interviews were conducted during phase 1 of the study. The nurses' phase 1 interview schedule incorporates key themes and concepts derived from the literature, which provide the framework through which the main theoretical aspects of the study are explored. This chapter reports the findings from the staff nurses' phase 1 interviews and incorporates a number of major themes, each of which is described in turn. These include the effects on nursing staff of having relatives around the ward, the range of demands that are made on nurses' time and personal resources, communications between relatives and staff, the nurses' experiences of stress, their coping responses and their perceived needs for support. The main themes to emerge from analysis of the staff nurses' phase 1 interviews are summarized in Table 5.2.

Table 5.2: Themes and subthemes in the staff nurses' accounts

Relatives around the ward	Effect on workload
	Basic hospitalities
Competing demands	Fighting fires
	Nurses under siege
Staff/relative contact	Negotiating the minefield
	Barriers and channels
Professional issues	Knowing our limits
	Nurses as advocates
Stress and coping	Sources and symptoms
	Coping strategies
	Nurses grieve too
	Support needs of nurses
Education and training	Pre-registration experience
	Post-registration provision
	Need for more training

Thematic analysis

Relatives around the ward

The nurses described the effects on staff and on the ward routine when a dying patient's relatives stayed around the ward for extended periods of time. Most agreed that it did add to the general workload, and several nurses also indicated that the relatives' presence created a sense of discomfort and unease in the staff. The following quotes illustrate the nurses' views in relation to this theme.

> I know it sounds terrible, but if you're really busy, the relative being there puts you under a lot more pressure.
>
> Interview no. 9

> You can't just ignore them, you've got to offer them cups of tea and talk to them, and make sure they're comfy in their chair, and ask is there anything they need.
>
> Interview no. 13

> It makes you very aware of what you say and what you do. You've got to sort of find corners yourself to discuss the things that you might do more openly if they weren't around.
>
> Interview no. 11

You've got to be more careful, more sensitive at the nurses' station. If the patients are in a bed that's opposite the nurses' station . . . . If the nurses are maybe having a carry-on or something, they've to keep their voices down and behave a bit better.

Interview no. 13

The nurses were emphatic and unanimous in their judgements about what they perceived to be the relatives' unmet needs for access to facilities for privacy, comfort and rest. Revealing insights into the nurses' feelings about this situation are provided in the following exemplars.

They need a room where they could sit and talk among themselves just to get away. Some people sit all day and all night and it's very stressful because there's nowhere for them to go.

Interview no. 9

A relatives' room – we desperately need one. They should have somewhere private especially if they're staying overnight. Somewhere to go and put their head down for a couple of hours, just to give them privacy to collect their thoughts.

Interview no. 14

We have no room for them to go and sit in and have a cup of tea or anything like that. They can stay overnight if they want to although they've got nothing but a chair to sit on.

Interview no. 13

As the dying patient's condition deteriorated and death approached, the nurses acknowledged that the relatives' needs for support from staff escalated. However, more than half of the nurses' sample expressed reservations about the extent to which they felt those needs were currently being met.

The relatives need to know that there's someone there that will respond to them. Someone they can turn to. Whether it's just to chat generally or just somebody to be there. And we're not geared towards that in here. It's a terrible thing to say, but we just don't have the time. It's awful.

Interview no. 11

They need contact with the nursing staff, they need information and they need that repeated and they also need privacy, somewhere to withdraw and get away.

Interview no. 12

Competing demands

A very strong and compelling theme in the data was represented by perceived lack of time and the range of competing demands on the nurses' time and resources that prevented them from delivering the level of care that the dying patient's relatives required. Frequent and recurring references were made to these difficulties, the most frequently expressed concerns being the demands posed by the pace and activity level in the wards and sheer pressure of time. The quotes below graphically illustrate the nurses' dilemma and the distress that this can generate.

> If there's someone lying acutely ill in the next bed, where do I divide my time? Do I sit with this relative who's just been told very bad news or do I deal with this acutely ill patient? We're not exactly over-endowed with staff in the ward.
>
> Interview no. 3

> Other demands might make you avoid going to a relative. Not because you don't want to deal with them, but because you know at the back of your head that there are so many other things to do.
>
> Interview no. 7

> All his wife wanted to do was sit and have a wee chat and I found myself squinting at my watch, because I had a drug round to do at 5 o'clock. It's dreadful. I wanted to be there for her. I really did. She just wanted to talk . . . she didn't want answers. And here I was squinting at my watch thinking 'if I don't get this drug round done now, there's going to be this delay or that delay.' Then I thought 'that's dreadful, this could be that man's last day on earth and I'm worrying about a drug round'. But there was just me, an auxiliary and a student and I had to leave her. You shouldn't have to do that. I felt so bad.
>
> Interview no. 11

Clarke (1984) described stress as an imbalance between demand and coping. These data confirm that nurses experience stress as a result of excessive and competing demands, coupled with inadequate resources to support their coping efforts. Avoidance tactics alluded to in the above exemplars represent defensive coping strategies already described in the stress and coping literature, and also highlighted in literature relating to the care of dying patients and their families (Folkman 1984; Maguire 1985a; Wilkinson 1991; Fallowfield 1993b).

Staff–relative contact

Staff–relative contact was clearly a difficult area for the staff nurses. With just one exception the nurses admitted feeling hesitant about approaching the dying patient's family. Several reasons for this were reported. The nurses expressed concerns about their own ability to deal with emotionally charged encounters and about the limited freedom they believed that they had to answer questions put to them by the patients' relatives.

> I think nurses sometimes . . . ehm use the excuse of it having to be the medical staff who discuss diagnosis . . . to sort of fob relatives off. But it *is* awkward. It's difficult talking about cancer. It's the word everyone shies away from . . . cancer and dying and stuff like that. And so nurses won't talk to the relative about it, they'll just say 'a doctor's got to speak to you about it'.
>
> Interview no. 14

> You feel that it's maybe the doctor that should speak to them but at that late stage you don't want to say, 'I should really get the doctor to speak to you about that'. Sometimes you feel 'I should really just talk to you'. But then you worry about saying the right things, or saying too much. You know? . . . Is it my *place* to be saying this?
>
> Interview no. 11

Communicating with relatives was reported as particularly stressful when nurses didn't know what the family had already been told about the patient's prognosis, and in situations where relatives did not want the diagnosis to be disclosed to the patient. The stress generated by such situations is evident in the quotes below.

> There's been circumstances where the wife doesn't want the husband to know the diagnosis, and the husband doesn't want the wife to know. And we are running in circles round each other. And you are frightened to open your mouth in case you put your foot in it. That's one of the worst things.
>
> Interview no. 10

> It puts an awful lot of stress on the patient and on the relative . . . *and on the nurse.* Because the patient *knows.* In themselves they know. And you're trying to tell the relatives that, but they would rather have the patient in ignorant bliss. [sounds annoyed] And they are building up all these barriers and the patient is sitting there really worried . . . and not able to talk things through.
>
> Interview no. 12

The language used by the nurses to describe their contact with families highlighted the uneasy relationship that seemed to exist between nurses and relatives. The text was liberally peppered with 'combat' metaphors suggesting that nurses to some extent felt 'under siege'. Examples of these metaphors include 'we're in the firing line', 'it's like walking through a minefield', 'you'd get shot down in flames', 'it could all blow up in your face' and 'you're ducking round corners diving for cover'. Further evidence of this tension is demonstrated in the following exemplars.

> They sometimes question the care which is being given and that is obviously kind of stressful. The whole experience is stressful because of the emotional commitment you have to put into it.
>
> Interview no. 3

> Sometimes relatives can actually be quite stroppy and they can throw up a barrier. It just depends on the individual. Families as a whole can be quite awkward. Always questioning what you're doing, and it seems as if they're slighting your nursing. And I think nurses take umbrage at that. I certainly have.
>
> Interview no. 3

Most of the nurses understood that relatives feel hesitant about approaching staff. Various reasons for the relatives' hesitancy were suggested and some of the approach strategies that relatives employ were described.

> If the ward is looking extremely busy and the nurses are looking harassed, I think a lot of the relatives are put off by that and are reluctant to come and speak to you. In case we think that they're being a nuisance.
>
> Interview no. 4

> The relatives just tend to stand in the corridor until you pass by and then they try to grab your attention. Or they hang about outside the room . . . hovering . . . looking for somebody . . . or if you're sitting at the desk a lot of them come up to the desk.
>
> Interview no. 1

Interprofessional issues

A range of issues relating to aspects of interprofessional communication were raised. It was strikingly evident that this area posed problems for most of the nurses. As previously reported, difficulties were experienced when nurses felt handicapped in their freedom to respond to relatives' questions. Around half of the nurses voiced concerns about this and, as the exemplars below show, a sense of professional impotence emerged from the data.

> It's very much only the caring, the basic caring needs that nurses can give information about. Anything above that or more than that it's got to be the doctor.
>
> Interview no. 6

> Yes I think there are restrictions placed upon us. Certain questions . . . not that I'm not *qualified* to answer, because of course I am . . . but I think are best left to medical staff. I mean I wouldn't dream of telling them the outcome of tests. I think that's something that should be dealt with by medical staff.
>
> Interview no. 11

The data reveal tacitly recognized spheres of professional responsibility within which nurses and doctors operate in relation to the transmission of information. This causes problems for nurses, several of whom expressed a wish to be included, or at least informed, when information is being relayed to relatives. Nurses indicated that they would feel better equipped to support the family if they knew the relatives' current understanding and acceptance of the patient's condition.

> I think that everybody should be spoken to with a nurse there, so that you would know exactly what has been said.
>
> Interview no. 1

> A lot of the time, the doctors haven't even come to you and kept you a 100 per cent up to date with the treatment of a particular patient. So, if the relative comes to you in the meantime . . . you don't have the information.
>
> Interview no. 1

Stress, coping and support

Using a 4-point Likert scale, the nurses were asked to rate the level of stress that they experienced when dealing with the dying patient's family from 'not stressful at all', 'slightly stressful', 'fairly stressful' or 'very stressful'. All but one rated this aspect of care as either 'very stressful' (7) or 'fairly stressful' (10). One opted for 'slightly stressful' and no one selected 'not stressful at all'.

Sources of stress

A range of factors that generate stress in nurses caring for the dying patient's family was reported. It has already been established that competing demands within the ward cause stress to nurses. Difficulties with interprofessional communication and having to field 'difficult' questions, which the nurses felt ill-equipped to answer, also resulted in stress. A number of nurses also reported stress caused by witnessing the relatives' emotional responses – especially their anger. The diverse origins of the nurses' stress is revealed below.

> It is *very* difficult to cope with. Particularly if the ward is really busy and you are maybe having a bad day or whatever. And it's difficult when someone's being aggressive towards you and you have to try and placate them. It is a very stressful thing to do you know . . . and having to keep calm yourself.
>
> Interview no. 5

> Seeing them when it's obviously somebody that they care so much about. To see them sitting watching their husband dying. You can see the pain in their eyes.
>
> Interview no. 5

> What I hate most is handing over the patient's clothing in a plastic bag. There's got to be a better way to do this. Because it just looks awful. I find it all quite difficult . . . . Seeing how the relatives react . . . it's all very difficult.
>
> Interview no. 13

The stigma of stress

The data suggest that, although all of the nurses had reported that they felt under stress, few would openly admit it because they believed that this might cause negative judgements to be made about them. The following quote illustrates the social pressure, which nurses can feel under, to deny or conceal their stress.

> I don't think anybody does admit to it. It's not something you come in and say, 'Oh, I was really stressed' or 'I found it really hard to cope with that situation' because you don't hear anybody else saying it. You don't see anyone else cracking up under the strain.
>
> Interview no. 7

Coping strategies

The range of coping strategies reported by the nurses reveals evidence of the emotion-focused and problem-focused strategies previously described in the literature (Wrubel et al. 1981; Clarke 1984; Folkman 1984; Lazarus 1985). The data confirm that emotion-focused strategies were used liberally by virtually all the respondents. The strategies that they reported, with the frequency with which they were used indicated in brackets, included talking to family and colleagues (16), getting away from the situation (5), drinking alcohol (9), smoking (3), physical activity or exercise (2), and relaxation or aromatherapy (2).

Emotion-focused (palliative) strategies, while not dealing with the stress at source, are geared towards helping individuals to feel better, albeit temporarily, thus making the stressful experience more bearable. The exemplars below offer illustrative examples of the strategies nurses' use in their 'palliative' approaches to coping.

> When I go home I rant and rave. I just let it all come out. And I go out socializing, or out for a meal . . . just to stay away from it . . . . And I go out for the odd drink. But mainly I just talk . . . . Constantly. When I went home the other day after my shift, poor Joe's ears were burning. He listened to me for three solid hours.
>
> Interview no. 10

> More often than not I'll just go away into my room and shut the door. I just don't want to be disturbed. I also find, believe it or not, that housework helps. It gets rid of all this pent up energy inside you.
>
> Interview no. 14

> I've taken up aromatherapy. Sometimes I have problems sleeping so I got into using aromatherapy and callanetics and watching TV. Anything to just relax . . . I don't smoke. I do drink but I don't drink if I'm working the next day.
>
> Interview no. 13

Problem-focused strategies are specifically aimed at modifying or removing the stress at source. Such strategies were very much less in evidence in the nurses' accounts, but examples of problem-focused strategies that did emerge included assessing workload priorities and delegating work to others. Only two respondents reported using such strategies and they reserved these for such 'exceptional' circumstances as described below.

> When I'm really stressed, I try and delegate some of the things I have to do to other members of staff to take some of the pressure off myself. There comes a stage when I think 'I just can't possibly do all this'.
>
> Interview no. 10

The transactional nature of the nurses' stress and their coping responses were clearly apparent in the data. The relative paucity of problem-focused coping behaviours suggest that nurses feel unable to influence the demands that are made on them and may also explain their heavy reliance on 'palliative', emotion-focused coping efforts. The data leave little doubt that nurses experience significant stress with this aspect of their practice. Indeed, in the course of the current analysis stress has been an overarching theme which has pervaded virtually every part of the analysis. The high emotional cost that nurses pay for their commitment to this aspect of care has been widely reported in the literature (Ceslowitz 1989; McGrath, Reid and Boore 1989; Nash 1989) and is encapsulated in a few words by a young staff nurse:

> You get involved with the patient and involved with their relatives and you start getting to know them . . . and they get to know you . . . and it all becomes so painful and hard.
>
> Interview no. 7

Nurses grieve too

The pain so graphically described above offers a reminder that professional carers also experience grief within the context of their personal and professional life. It has already been reported in the literature that the death of very young patients elicits particularly strong feelings of distress in nurses (Harper and Fulton 1977; Fisher 1988; Ceslowitz 1989). This was confirmed in the current study in which the nurses also reported severe stress where a sense of identification had developed with a dying patient, perhaps of similar age or with a family with a similar structure and background to their own.

The exemplar below offers insight into feelings generated in such situations.

> A few weeks ago we had a young 24-year-old die in the ward. That was the most difficult thing I have ever had to deal with in my whole career. It was hard

watching her mother and her two brothers suffer. I couldn't switch myself off from that. I was going home at night and that was just in my head all of the time. That was really, really hard.

Interview no. 1

Feelings of loss also tended to be influenced by such factors as the duration and frequency of the contact that the nurse had had with that particular patient and family. Nurses can undoubtedly form close attachments with patients who have been in the ward for some time and the feelings of personal loss that can be experienced on the death of such patients are described below.

They say you're not supposed to get emotionally involved but if you're nursing somebody for such a long time you feel as if you're part of their lives. A very big part towards the end and it is very, very hard.

Interview no. 7

The price that this level of emotional involvement exacts is vividly described by the young staff nurse quoted below.

I couldn't even speak to my husband about it because I was so upset. And he hadn't a clue what was wrong with me. He kept saying, 'You'll have to tell me' . . . so he could help me. And I *couldn't*. I was like this [weeping]. The worst part of it was I was going on holiday the next day. She died the next morning . . . and I was going on *holiday* . . .

Interview no. 1

Although it was believed to be 'theoretically' acceptable to show emotions about a patient's death, the reality was judged to be different. Several nurses reported that they felt that there was an expectation that they should 'put on a brave face' and that failure to do this might elicit disapproval from others and engender personal feelings of inadequacy in themselves.

I suppose you shouldn't feel ashamed or guilty about crying. You really shouldn't. But sometimes it's expected that nurses should just cope with everything that's thrown at them but they shouldn't show their own emotions.

Interview no. 1

Feelings of discomfort experienced when dealing with grieving people seemed to be intensified when a nurse was also coping with personal grief. Three nurses spontaneously described their personal experiences of loss and how this affected their ability to cope with care of the dying patient and family. One nurse's personal vulnerability is vividly revealed in the following exemplar. Metaphors in the language she used convey strong images of unhealed wounds and of her feeling engulfed by the relatives' pain and grief.

> I can't cope with their pain because it's overflowing into me . . . It's all still very raw inside me [personal grief] and their pain brings it back to me. I'm sorry but I just can't separate it. Their pain overflows into me and I find the whole experience just as painful for me as it is for them.
>
> Interview no. 11

Support for staff

The nurses, without exception, reported the supportive benefits of talking to ward colleagues and peers, and of having a supportive person outside work to confide in, usually a partner or parent, who would listen sympathetically to their concerns and feelings. The exemplar reveals the support network reportedly used by many of the respondents.

> Well, there's your colleagues. And out of work good old Mum's always on hand. She'll ask you when you come in from work what sort of day did you have and such like. But actually going to an outsider maybe like a friend and just talking about it and them giving you a sympathetic ear. That helps . . . it really does.
>
> Interview no. 14

Strong views were expressed about the quality and nature of the support that the nurses believed was available to them within the work situation. Apart from the previously reported benefits of peer support, responses were overwhelmingly negative, and the nurses generally perceived a lack of support and concern by management. An example of such views is offered below.

> The 'powers that be' . . . . It's *nothing* to them. The girls in the ward might say to you 'away you go and have a seat and we'll deal with this'. But that's at ward level – never outwith.
>
> Interview no. 3

However, one nurse reported a very positive experience. She describes being supported by her nurse manager when, as a newly

qualified staff nurse, she had to deal with the parents of a child who
had died in the ward.

> The Nursing Officer in that ward was great. She said to me, 'I know you have
> just finished your training and I know you are going to have to deal with these
> relatives' and then she turned round and said to me 'It's OK if you cry.' You
> know nobody had ever said that to me before.
>
> Interview no. 14

The manager's acknowledgement of this nurse's essential human-
ity and associated needs was clearly appreciated. The nurse
recounted this incident some 5 years after the event. A number of
nurses also suggested that they would gain support from a greater
degree of interprofessional collaboration and from access to additional education and training relevant to this area of practice.

Nurse education

With just one exception the nurses expressed dissatisfaction with their
basic educational preparation for terminal care in terms of its adequacy
and relevance to practice. Pre-registration education for all but one of
the nurses had been within colleges of nursing. One nurse had taken an
undergraduate course in nursing studies in a university and she alone
expressed satisfaction with her preparation for this aspect of practice.
The comments offered below are strongly representative of the nurses'
views about their educational preparation in this area.

> I don't think our basic training prepared us at all. I mean you might have stuff
> written down on paper and it might all make sense but experience is the only
> way you learn these things.
>
> Interview no. 10

> Maybe if they [teachers] had talked more about the relatives and the problems that
> they might have. All you could think about was the patient and washing their face
> and making sure they don't have pressure sores. The relatives rarely came into it.
>
> Interview no. 9

Paradoxically, although the nurses were openly critical about
their previous educational experiences, they unanimously and
repeatedly appealed for access to further training, especially in the
fields of communication and counselling.

> We really should be trained properly in counselling skills. I've only been quali-
> fied a short while and you can be sort of anxious about whether you're going to
> put your foot in it and upset them.
>
> Interview no. 2

> I would really like to do some sort of counselling course. You just never ever
> know what to say to patients' relatives.
>
> Interview no. 11

Adopting the mantle of staff nurse proved a traumatic transition for some. The quotes below reveal the feelings that this role change can engender.

> I thought I would be led in by the hand and that was just not the case. The first
> day I was in charge I knew nothing. *Nothing*. Nobody said I was going to feel that
> inadequate. The only way I got through was by experience.
>
> Interview no. 3

> I've only been qualified a short time and you can be sort of anxious about
> whether you're going to put your foot in it and upset them.
>
> Interview no. 2

Several nurses, as illustrated below, expressed the view that the type of skills needed to offer support around the time of death were most often acquired within the practice setting by role modelling on others and by gaining experience. Advantages of these approaches to learning are highlighted below.

> In the clinical areas you saw at a glance how qualified staff coped with speaking
> to relatives. Both the good and the bad points.
>
> Interview no. 7

> One staff nurse I thought was really good. She was able to approach relatives
> and say, 'I want to have a wee chat with you . . .'. And I thought at that time,
> 'God, I'll never, ever be able to go up to somebody and say anything like that.'
> But I remember her, just her manner and the way she was.
>
> Interview no. 10

> Death is one of these things that happen to us all eventually and people are kind
> of too frightened to face it. You would need something [course] which helps
> people to express themselves. That helps them to open up and talk about it.
>
> Interview no. 10

Needs for more effective dissemination of information and for improved access to post-registration courses were unanimously expressed. Comments were also made about the difficulties that the nurses experienced in trying to secure funding and study leave to attend relevant courses and study days.

Conclusion

These data reveal examples of nurses' insight and sensitivity to the needs of the dying patient's family. The data also reveal that nurses experience significant stress associated with this aspect of care.

This stress was found to be generated by a range of factors, including the emotionally charged character of the situation, the competing and pressing demands that are made on nurses' time and resources, and the lack of facilities and resources for the support of relatives, and by the nature of the relationships and practices that operate within health-care teams.

The nurses' and the relatives' phase 1 data reported above were presented by the researcher at the start of a 2-day workshop. The nurses then used these data to design clinical standards for care and support for the dying patient's family. Processes involved in this initiative, and during subsequent implementation of the standards, are reported in Chapter 6.

Chapter 6
The intervention

This chapter describes the intervention phase of the study which represented a period of several months of intensive effort for the participating nurses. It also explains how the intervention was developed, the work that the participating nurses undertook in the study wards and the ways in which the intervention was monitored and evaluated. Some of the decisions that were taken about the choice of the intervention approach, and the issues that were involved in implementing a planned change initiative as part of a research study, are discussed with reference to the relevant literature.

Selection of the intervention

Experiential workshop

The decision to incorporate an experiential workshop was mainly influenced by the researcher's previous professional experience of facilitating such initiatives, but was also supported by evidence from the literature (Faulkner 1988a). Experiential approaches have been found to be particularly appropriate for exploring attitudes and for developing interpersonal skills, especially in relation to terminal care (Hurtig and Stewin 1990; Baynton-Lees 1993). This decision was reinforced by the phase 1 data which offered evidence of the staff nurses' needs for opportunities to improve their communication skills.

The decision to restrict the workshop to 2 days was guided by resource implications. Although a longer course of study would have been preferred, 2 days was the maximum period of time that the nurse managers were able to release the nurses from their clinical duties. The length of the workshop was further influenced by the fact that the researcher had to negotiate funding for agency nurses to provide replacement cover for the period that the nurses would be absent from their wards.

It was judged important to conduct the workshop within the university setting because this would enable the staff nurses physically to withdraw from the acute hospital situation and move into an academic environment for a brief period of intensive learning. It was also hoped that, by basing the initiative within an academic setting, the joint practice and theoretical elements of the change initiative that the nurses would be engaged in would be underscored.

Quality assurance framework

As described in Chapter 4, a quality assurance framework was selected for implementing an evaluated intervention because it was judged likely that the nurses would be familiar with the idea of standard setting. Employing a standard-setting approach would also allow the intervention to be developed by those most directly responsible for its implementation. This 'bottom-up' approach to implementing change has been found to be important for engendering ownership in and commitment to a change initiative and could therefore increase its potential for success (Kitson 1986; Harvey 1994). Finally, standard setting was judged to have merit because the approach encourages nurses to reflect on their own practice and to conduct ongoing evaluations of the care that they deliver (Methot et al. 1992).

The workshop

After phase 1 of the study, the staff nurses attended a 2-day workshop conducted in the university where the researcher was based. Within the limits imposed by the predetermined aims of the workshop (see pp. 124–6), the structure and content of the workshop were largely negotiated and therefore the programme was drawn up retrospectively.

The researcher formally opened the workshop and presented the findings from the analysis of the nurses' and the relatives' phase 1 interviews. Thereafter, to reduce the risk of bias, the researcher withdrew and the remainder of the workshop was conducted by two appropriately qualified independent facilitators.

The decision to have the workshop conducted by external facilitators rather than by the researcher was taken within the context of the original evaluation research design, and stemmed from concern that the validity of the study might have been threatened if the evaluator was also to be involved in the development and implementation of an intervention.

The distance between the researcher and participants, and the control and objectivity that this philosophical stance implies, eventually presented both practical and philosophical problems for the researcher. These tensions are explored further later in this chapter.

Developing the standards

With the nurses working in small groups, the phase 1 results were discussed and, from these discussions, the participants identified key issues that they believed needed to be addressed when developing standards for their own wards. The list below represents the range of issues that emerged from the nurses' feedback and thus represents areas collectively judged to be of concern to nurses and families.

Areas addressed in the standards

- Relatives' access to comfortable, private accommodation
- Relatives' access to a named nurse with knowledge of the patient's prognosis and treatment, and the relatives' current level of understanding and acceptance
- Relatives' access to other members of the care team
- Interprofessional communication and record keeping
- Family support and information around the time of death
- Relatives' access to spiritual support and support agencies.

From this list the nurses decided which areas they felt they could address within their own ward. The workshop facilitators then delivered a broadly theoretical overview of quality assurance and of standard setting using the Dynamic Standard Setting System (DySSSy) approach (Harvey 1994).

During the remainder of the workshop the nurses worked in two groups, each group supported by a facilitator. Self-selection resulted in the emergence of hospital-specific groups and interesting differences emerged in the areas addressed in the standards. Within each 'hospital-specific group', further differences emerged between wards, thus generating truly local standards. Although some nurses decided that their priorities should centre on introducing the 'Named Nurse' for the family and other communication initiatives, others opted to invest most of their energies into securing improvements in facilities for relatives. Neither the workshop facilitators nor the researcher made any attempt to influence the nurses' decisions about which areas they chose to address in their standards.

In keeping with the predetermined workshop aims (see pp. 124–6), the final half-day of the workshop was entirely devoted to addressing the nurses' own specific concerns. Each group worked with a facilitator and the content and approach were negotiated. Although the programme reveals slight differences in emphasis, both groups elected to focus on the difficulties that nurses experience when interacting with dying patients and their families, and on measures to manage the stress that they experience with this aspect of their practice.

Apart from the data feedback session, and the subsequent theoretical session on quality assurance and standard setting, an experiential approach was adopted throughout the workshop because such an approach has been found to encourage participants to examine their attitudes and to share feelings and experiences (Hurtig and Stewin 1990; Baynton-Lees 1993).

Evaluating the intervention

At the time of the workshop, the researcher was still working within the evaluation research method and was committed to the principles of illuminative evaluation (Parlett and Hamilton 1972; Gallego 1987; Guba and Lincoln 1989; Powers and Knapp 1995). It has already been reported in Chapter 4 that illuminative evaluation focuses not just on outcomes, but also on the process of a change initiative, and the approach typically draws on data from a range of sources and uses qualitative approaches that allow the participants' perspective to be sought (Gallego 1987; Powers and Knapp 1995).

The decision was made to conduct the workshop evaluation 3 months after the workshop was taken because, at this juncture, the nurses should be able to provide an overall evaluation of the intervention processes. The evaluation could then seek views about participating in the workshop and elicit their experiences when facilitating the development and implementation of standards in their wards.

Although the main approach to evaluating the intervention would take the form of a comparative analysis of the nurses' and the relatives' phase 1 and phase 2 interview data, it was also judged important to provide an evaluation strategy that focused on the nurses' experiences of the workshop and the post workshop activities while those experiences were still recent or indeed current. It was also judged important to provide a vehicle for the nurses to express their views anonymously. For these reasons, a questionnaire was developed and was sent to each nurse, together with a stamped addressed envelope for its return. The participants were given assurances of confidentiality and anonymity.

The questionnaire contained a mixture of closed and open questions. Space was provided for comments. The instrument had two main parts, each containing a number of sections. The first part sought the nurses' views about the 2-day workshop. The second part focused on the nurses' experiences during the post workshop period when they were facilitating the development and implementation of the standards.

A very brief account of the nurses' responses is given below. Evaluation data that focus on the workshop are reported. Collated evaluation data that focus on the *post workshop* period are reported later in this chapter after the researcher's account of the intervention period. The decision to report the evaluation data in this way represents an effort to preserve a coherent and chronological flow in the account.

Collated evaluation of the workshop

The first part of the questionnaire sought the nurses' views about the workshop and was organized into several sections. Headings from these sections are used to present the collated evaluation data.

The learning approach

Data reveal that the nurses found the experiential approach to be appropriate for meeting their learning needs and for providing a supportive learning environment. All the comments were very positive in this area as this sample of the nurses' views confirm.

Very skilled facilitators – the counselling sessions were very helpful.

I learned a lot about myself, my colleagues and relatives' feelings.

Participation was an excellent learning method.

The workshop atmosphere made it easy to raise issues and emotions without feeling like a failure.

Length and pace of the workshop

Just over half the respondents indicated that they would have appreciated having longer than 2 days for the workshop, several stating that this had resulted in a faster pace than they would otherwise have preferred. However, almost half judged the pace to be 'just about right'. The nurses' expressed these views as follows:

We had to move quickly as we had only two days. It would have been better if we had longer and could have taken things more slowly.

The facilitators were excellent, well experienced, paced it expertly.

We knew our time limits and just knuckled down.

Achievement of workshop aims

The participants unanimously judged that all four workshop aims had been met. As a large number of comments were offered in relation to each of these aims, only a very brief sample is provided below.

Aim 1: to provide feedback on the phase 1 interview data

More than half the respondents indicated that they would have liked more time for the data feedback. However, all the comments confirmed that the nurses had enjoyed hearing the phase 1 findings. Some claimed to have found the relatives' data to be 'quite shocking' and 'very moving'.

Aim 2: to provide an overview of quality assurance and standard setting

This was judged by all but one of the participants to have been successfully achieved. Evaluation data reveal that the nurses appreciated the approach adopted. The formal teaching session had provided the background knowledge needed for the more active sessions on standard setting that followed. The extent to which the nurses' needs were met in relation to this aim is revealed in the comments below.

> Yes – this was very much achieved, good explanations and a lot of time spent on this.
>
> This was my first experience of standard setting and it has proven to be most valuable.
>
> Between the workshop and the support I have had from R since the workshop I feel I have learned a great deal about quality assurance and standard setting.
>
> Never having set standards before I felt a little bit lost at times.

Aim 3: to use the data to create standards for improved family care

In terms of workshop activity, this aim was considered to have been largely achieved. However, most of the detailed standard-setting activity took place during the post workshop period and, at the 3-month post workshop evaluation stage, energetic efforts to complete the implementation process were still under way in most of the wards. The following quote supports this finding:

> We are still trying to get our standard ratified but the workshop did give us an excellent start.

Aim 4: to address issues raised by the nurses during their interviews

This aim was judged to have been satisfactorily achieved. Comments revealed that the stress management and counselling input had been appreciated. The data suggest that the nurses had also valued the opportunity that the workshop presented to ventilate their anxieties and to give and receive support.

> All the nurses benefited from sharing feelings.
>
> It was an ideal opportunity to express our views and get things off our chests.
>
> The whole workshop could easily have been spent on this but we did cover it significantly.

What was liked most?

When asked what they had liked *most* about the workshop, eight responses related to hearing the research data and six nurses rated the sessions on counselling skills as their top choice. Frequent comments were also made about the benefits of meeting the other nurses in the study, and the friendliness and skill of the workshop facilitators. A number of very specific responses related to the facilitative and sharing climate that was generated at the workshop as the following quotes reveal:

> I found the whole experience quite moving. We developed close bonds with strangers very quickly.

> I liked the fact that there was not a lot of note taking and we could share ideas and issues.

> I could express emotions most of which I did not realize, or want to realize, that I had.

> It wasn't until I talked about an experience that I realized how much I had been affected by it.

> The feeling of doing something positive. There is too much 'putting down' in nursing nowadays.

> We felt we were going back to our wards able to make good changes.

What was liked least?

When asked what they had liked *least* about the workshop, the nurses' comments were far fewer and those that were offered focused mainly on issues such as the room size or the uncomfortable chairs. Almost half commented that there had not been anything that they had not liked during the workshop. However, two respondents did suggest that they had not liked the time constraints that the length of the workshop had imposed, and one of these two stated that she would have preferred a more structured teaching approach.

This concludes the nurses' evaluation of the workshop activities and experiences. Data from the second part of evaluation focus on the *post workshop* period. The nurses' collated post workshop evaluation data follow the researcher's account of the intervention.

Part 2 of the intervention

Implementing the standards

Implementation of the standards took place over a period of several months. The nurses left the workshop with an outline of the areas that they planned to address in their wards, and with newly acquired knowledge about quality assurance and standard setting. They began by discussing the standard outline drawn up at the workshop with the ward nursing teams. It has already been established that, in the Donabedian model for standard setting, 'structure' criteria encompass the range of resources, facilities and documentation systems needed to meet the agreed standard (Harvey 1994). Once all the nurses had agreed that the standard should be developed as a ward initiative, the difficult process began of putting the changes needed to meet the structure criteria into place.

During this post workshop period the staff nurses, now acting as facilitators within their own ward teams, were involved in extensive liaison with others, including ward sisters/charge nurses, the nursing team on day and night duty, nurse managers, medical colleagues, chaplains and social workers. Some even contacted builders, estate managers and various charities in their efforts either to provide a relatives' room where none had previously existed or/and to obtain comfortable furnishings and equipment for existing rooms. In several wards the 'Named Nurse' initiative was successfully implemented and this principle of care was extended to relatives of very ill or dying patients. In two wards, interdisciplinary meetings were convened by the staff nurse facilitators to discuss ways to improve communication between staff and the dying patients' relatives, and to find ways to improve interprofessional communication.

At various stages the facilitators contacted nurse managers for consultation or to seek approval or support for new developments. In one of the hospitals the quality assurance nurse was very actively supportive of the research initiative and she made herself available to provide advice for the nurses during the standard development period. When the final draft was accepted by all, the standards were sent with their monitoring and evaluation tools to the Unit Nurse in each hospital for ratification.

The methodological shift

Securing the changes in facilities and practice required to meet the standard criteria and developing the standard from a rough outline to the stage of ratification proved to be a slow and often frustrating process, during which the nurses required a considerable degree of support. During this time, the researcher was increasingly drawn into the process and as a consequence the distance between the researcher and the participating nurses steadily closed. The nature and level of the researcher's involvement during the intervention period are fully detailed below. In the researcher's judgement, the standard development and implementation processes are unlikely to have been successfully completed without this external support.

It was becoming evident that the original evaluation design was no longer sustainable. This shift did not represent a particular moment in time, but was rather a growing realization that the study was evolving in response to the dynamic and reflexive influences within the research environment, as a result of which practical, ethical and philosophical issues had to be addressed.

Ethically there were a number of considerations. First, the researcher was accountable to the funding body that had agreed to support the work on the strength of its potential to benefit the quality of care provided in the study wards. Ethical approval had similarly been granted on the premise that the project was improvement oriented. The researcher also felt an ethical duty to the phase 1 relatives to ensure that the data they had contributed were used in the pursuit of enhanced care. The relatives had agreed to be interviewed during a difficult period in their lives. Altruism, often expressed as a wish to 'help others in the future', had motivated most of these relatives to participate in the study. Remaining distant from the participating nurses as they struggled with the difficulties of trying to implement change would also have felt, to the researcher, as if she were abandoning the nurses, especially given the effort that they had already invested in the study.

The dilemmas detailed above underscore the tension that can exist between the investigator's responsibility to the 'researched' and her responsibilities to science (Oiler Boyd 1993). In the current study, this was resolved by a decision to become actively associated with the participating nurses by providing them with mentorship and support, but to do this from outside the action setting.

The researcher's main point of contact in the study wards was with the participating staff nurses rather than with the whole nursing team. It was judged that, in this way, fidelity to the spirit of the 'bottom-up' approach could still be maintained and the potential for success of the change initiative, and the empowerment of the nurses, could be maximized (Harvey 1994). Practical considerations also influenced this decision. The size and the geographical spread of the study area, and the sheer numbers and diversity of staff that this involved, precluded a greater level of involvement of the researcher in the day-to-day activities of the ward teams associated with the change initiative.

Researcher's involvement in the intervention

Maintaining contact with the nurses

In the period following the workshop regular face-to-face and telephone contact was maintained with the staff nurse facilitators in the study wards. During ward visits the nurses discussed their progress and any problems encountered with the standard development and implementation procedures. A 'contact log' was maintained by the researcher to ensure that issues raised, progress made and difficulties encountered during this period were recorded. In this way a coherent account of events occurring across all eight study wards could be maintained.

Administrative support

Although it was judged important that the researcher did not directly influence the actual content of the standards, help was given with the layout of the standards, and the researcher also typed and modified these documents during various stages of their development. When the facilitators indicated that their ward teams were satisfied with the standard, the researcher designed monitoring and evaluation tools for use in each of the eight standards. One of the clinical standards, together with its evaluation tool, is given in Appendices 1 and 2.

Documentation systems

'Standard Evaluation Forms' were developed by the researcher for each individual ward's standard. Staff were asked to complete an evaluation for each family, to allow judgements to be made about the extent to which standard criteria were being met on an individual level. It was explained that these documents would also enable problems experienced by the staff using the standards to be identified and documented. A 'Record of Use Sheet' was also provided to enable the staff to monitor the overall frequency with which the standard was applied.

Feedback to the managers

During the intervention period, a series of meetings was arranged in both hospitals so that the senior nurses, including ward sisters/charge nurses, nurse managers, quality assurance nurses and unit nurses, could be provided with feedback and information. A phase 1 research report was produced for the managers which contained a synopsis of the phase 1 findings and information about the nature and conduct of the intervention that was currently taking place in their wards. It was hoped that these meetings would serve the combined role of providing information to the managers and establishing the researcher's role in supporting the staff nurses.

Feedback to the ward teams

An information pack was produced for each of the study wards. This pack described the aims and design of the study and offered an overview of the phase 1 research findings. Also included was a copy of the standard and evaluation tool developed for that particular ward and an explanation of the evaluation process that should be conducted. It was hoped that this level of dissemination might improve the ward teams' commitment to the initiative.

Production of a post workshop manual

Once all of the standards had been ratified, and the post workshop evaluation had been conducted, analysed and collated, a manual was produced for each participating nurse. The manual was intended to provide a means of consolidating the nurses' learning from the workshop, and it was also seen as a way of emphasizing the research-based nature of the work in which the nurses were currently involved. The manual contents included a brief review of the literature, an overview of the study design, results from the relatives' and nurses' phase 1 analysis, a copy of the workshop programme and a copy of the nurses' collated responses to the workshop evaluation. Copies of all eight clinical standards together with their evaluation tools were also included. Nineteen journal articles were included in the manual and these were reproduced with the kind permission of the copyright holders. Selection of these sources reflected issues raised by the nurses and relatives in the phase 1 interviews; the intention in providing this body of literature was to encourage further study and to promote evidence-based practice.

The above measures and activities were intended to provide practical, emotional and above all visible support for the staff nurses as they strove to secure the cooperation of their colleagues for the planned improvements in practice. The researcher's level of activity in the action setting during this intervention period, and the increasingly collaborative nature of the researcher–participant relationship, left little doubt that the study had evolved from an illuminative evaluation approach to an action research approach.

Nurses' evaluation of the post workshop period

Reports about the nurses' experiences were elicited during the researcher's regular visits to the wards. Field notes were made during this time using the contact log described above. These data and data collated from the post workshop evaluation confirm that this was a very demanding period, during which the nurses needed a considerable measure of support.

Post workshop evaluation data offer insight into the nurses' feelings and experiences during this intensive part of the study. The brief sections reported below represent the general areas explored in this part of the evaluation. An indication of how the nurses responded is also provided.

Support received

When asked 'what and who supported you during this period?', eight nurses named the researcher as their main source of support. Four reported that the ward sisters and other nurses on their ward had been very supportive, whereas several nurses found that having another staff nurse in the ward who could act as a 'partner' facilitator was very supportive. The quality assurance nurse in one hospital was also cited as a source of support by several nurses. The quotes below represent a sample of the views expressed.

> Both ward sisters offered a great deal of support and showed a lot of interest.
>
> [Researcher's] phone calls and visits were very much appreciated. She was a great support when needed.

> Having two staff nurses working together was good. We were both able to support each other.

Support lacking

When asked 'what support was needed but was lacking?', five of the nurses spoke about their difficulties in motivating other members of staff to work with them on the initiative. Three also expressed difficulties getting the ward sisters or managers to become involved. Unmet needs for support are evident in the quotes below.

> Ward staff are keen on the principle of the standard but they think that it's the facilitator alone who has to implement it and make it work.

> One sister was supportive but did not get actively involved; the other sister was antagonistic.

> Support was needed from nurse managers but not provided.

Success enjoyed

When asked to comment on the successes they had enjoyed during the intervention period, nine respondents described their 'greatest success' as getting the standard up and running. For two others, getting a relatives' room ready and furnished was reported as their main success. Nurses' feelings of achievement in these areas are illustrated below.

> Getting the standard ready and seeing it all typed up.

> I enjoyed learning about and drawing up the standard.

> I felt I had achieved a lot by getting the relatives' room ready.

Frustrations experienced

When asked to identify sources of frustration, four stated that they had no significant frustrations to report whereas six reported frustrations that came from a number of sources as the quotes below confirm.

> Time spent trying to motivate colleagues was frustrating.

> Waiting for other departments [builders] to act took so long.

> Time taken trying to get the room set up and the standard fully established.

Ward team's acceptance

When asked to comment on the level of acceptance by the ward team of the standard-setting initiative, eight comments, two negative and six positive, were received. The range of acceptance by ward staff is illustrated in the comments below.

> Fellow nurses on the ward thought the standard was great and are keen to raise funds for furniture for relatives' room.

> Acceptance was variable, some nit-picked but offered no constructive comments.

> Standard well accepted by the ward team who think it's been long overdue.

These evaluation data and observations, and field notes made during the intervention stage of the study, highlighted the complexity of the processes that the nurses and the researcher were collaboratively involved in. Although it was known at the outset that some form of educational intervention would be offered, the scale of change that this involved could not have been anticipated. Nor was the range and extent of the nurses' affective responses during and after the workshop anticipated. Thus, although the researcher had withdrawn from the workshop and from any involvement in the actual design of the intervention, it became increasingly clear as the study progressed that an important aspect of the researcher's role during the intervention phase of the study was to support the nurses through their experiences as they worked to facilitate change.

As the researcher was gradually drawn into the process, it also became clear that the extended participant–researcher relationship within a planned change initiative had caused the method to change to an action research approach which has its theoretical roots in change theory. As deeper understanding of the complex processes and relationships that were operating within the context of the study was sought, the literature was again consulted and this is reported. The reason why this literature is reported at this point is that it reflects an honest account of the course of the events that occurred in this study.

Action research

Action research is firmly based on change theory. It builds on people's motivation to change, provides them with the authority to make changes and offers them support and resources as they move towards change. Action research therefore represents a dynamic interaction between research and organizational change (Redfern and Norman 1990). Action research developed in response to dissatisfaction with the opposing philosophies of traditional quantitative–qualitative methods (Miles and Huberman 1984). The approach is heavily influenced by the work of Kurt Lewin, a social reformer, who explored issues such as racism and prison reform in post-war America (Lewin 1951; Hart and Bond 1995). As planned, change theory is so fundamental to the action research method that it is briefly summarized at this point before going on to consider action research theory in more detail (Bhola 1994; Lutjens and Tiffany 1994; Hagerman and Tiffany 1994).

Planned change models

Planned change models can be located on a continuum in relation to the level of external power that is exerted on the target group in order to effect change. Three commonly described models that can be placed along this continuum include the rational model, the normative model and the power-coercive model (Wright 1989).

The rational model

Rational models rely on low levels of external power and work best where there is universal readiness for change and the resistance to change is minimal (Tappen 1989). The rational model is described in three stages, beginning with the 'invention stage' where the leader identifies the need for change. This is followed by the 'diffusion stage' which involves getting the idea across to the group. In the final 'adoption stage' the change is implemented into practice. The newly adopted change then goes through a period of installation until it is 'institutionalized' into the system and becomes accepted practice (Tappen 1989). This model takes a holistic view of change, encourages an ethical use of power and enhances decision-making. It does, however, have limitations because it assumes a level of mutuality and equality not often evident in highly structured organizations such as health-care services (Bennis, Benne and Chin 1985; Broome 1990).

The 'power-coercive model'

This model occupies the opposite end of the continuum from the rational model, and it uses power and authority as a lever to effect change within a target system (Tappen 1989). It is neither participative nor democratic and is used mainly in situations where high levels of resistance are anticipated. Legal or social sanctions often operate to increase compliance. Such a model does have practical application, e.g. when enforcing regulations such as health and safety legislation, but it has clear limitations in most social structures (Tappen 1989).

Normative re-educative models

Normative models occupy the midpoint of the external power continuum and are largely based on Lewin's theory of planned change. Central to Lewin's theory is the notion that forces operate within a target system which facilitates change (driving forces) whereas other forces act to resist change (restraining forces). Study of these opposing forces, and their relative impact on the status quo, is called 'Force Field Analysis' (Broome 1990). Lewin's theory also describes the change process as occurring in three phases: 'unfreezing', 'moving' and 're-freezing'.

During the unfreezing stage the status quo is challenged and the need for change is acknowledged. Unfreezing takes time, is energy demanding and involves a period of psychological dissonance in those affected by the change. Dissonance is important because it generates the energy needed to reduce the mismatch between how things are now and how they ought to be. Provided that the organisational climate is appropriate, dissonance acts as an excellent motivator for change. The leader's role at the unfreezing stage is to introduce new information, encourage new behaviour, provide a supportive climate where anxieties can be ventilated and act as an energizer to overcome resistance (Mauksch and Miller 1981; Broome 1990; Elliott 1991).

During the movement stage that follows, complex negotiations and liaison may be involved as change processes are agreed, designed and implemented. Once change has occurred the final 're-freezing' stage aims to stabilize and integrate the changed state into the target system. During this stage, the leader continues to energize and reinforce the newly established behaviour but increasingly withdraws and delegates responsibility to others. The process of change is facilitated if a 'leverage' point can be identified in the target system. The lever might be a particular aspect of the system that is most easily affected, or a receptive individual or group that can provide the initial momentum for change. To this end, some planned change models incorporate a change agent to work with a target group as they seek to implement changes in practice (Havelock 1973; Lippitt 1973; Lathlean and Farnish 1984).

Normative models tend to be holistic, responsive and democratic in their orientation. These features render them philosophically congruent with the principles of action research (Broome 1990; Lutjens and Tiffany 1994). The main characteristics of normative change models are summarized below.

Normative planned change models (Schermerhorn 1981)

- Build change initiatives around a felt need
- Use sensitive methods to gather data to support the need for change
- Use effective communication skills to present the information to the target group
- Establish and maintain good interpersonal relationships throughout the period of change
- Use the personal charisma and influence of the leader to encourage participation within the group
- Provide assistance and support to the change agent.

Action research methods

Action research is conducted with people rather than on people. It is essentially a participative and problem-focused approach to implementing and evaluating change, and it encourages the implementation of research into practice and the evaluation of care (Greenwood 1984).

In action research, the relationship between theory and practice is interactive and dynamic and, as it encourages reflective practice, it has the potential to bring about fundamental changes in attitudes, beliefs and behaviour. As the approach is based on cooperation and collaboration, it also offers an appropriate vehicle for interprofessional enquiry provided that power relationships and role conflict issues are addressed before embarking on a study (Greenwood 1984; Titchen and Binnie 1993; Hart and Bond 1995). Akinsanya (1994) suggests that the case for research-based practice is now very strong and that any consideration of the theory–practice gap must acknowledge the relationship of knowledge to action. Action research does just that and it addresses some of the criticisms made about the value of traditional research approaches to nursing and the utility of the knowledge that they generate (Webb 1989).

Action research models

Models described for implementing change using action research include the 'insider model' and the 'outsider model' (Titchen and Binnie 1993). In the insider model a 'special' nurse, often with a research or other specialist background, is introduced into the study area in order to facilitate the process of change (Lathlean and Farnish 1984). In the outsider model a researcher, who is *not* part of the ward team, supports the staff as they work through the process of change (Webb 1989). In both models those who will implement and live with the change are closely involved in bringing it about. Although the insider model has greater potential for success, its limitations are that, of necessity, it is usually applied within a circumscribed research field. For change to be implemented over a wider area, an outsider model is usually deemed to be more appropriate (Broome 1990).

The researcher, in the outsider model, adopts the role of supporting, encouraging and, if possible, inspiring the people who are implementing the changes in practice. Risks in this model are that there will be failure of uptake or that early discontinuance of the change will occur. This is less likely to happen if those who implement the changes are closely involved in their design and if a sense of ownership in and commitment to the change initiative has developed (Titchen and Binnie 1993). Tensions can develop between the researcher and the 'actors' in the outsider model, especially if they do not share common values. Indeed the first stage in an action research study should be to establish the basic values that underpin the planned change. Also, the researcher has limited authority and, if the group fail to implement the change, or if they allow discontinuance, the researcher has limited powers to deal with this (Titchen and Binnie 1993).

Action research is democratic, collaborative and empowering. It explores problems within their situational and social context, thus giving research a firm base in reality (Greenwood 1984). By narrowing the distance between researcher and participants, it reduces the risk of research being seen as an esoteric, self-serving activity with limited relevance to practice (Elliott 1991).

Barriers to implementing action research

Social mores, traditions and internal belief systems can operate as constraints to implementing research findings in practice. Also, if research sets out merely to criticize practitioners, it is doomed to failure (Redfern and Norman 1990). Ways in which findings are communicated can restrict their potential for impact on practice, and research reports are often inaccessible to practitioners or are presented in ways that are unpalatable and difficult to read (Basset 1992). Furthermore, conflicts can surface between managers and practitioners which might inhibit collaborative efforts and reduce the chances of success of an action research initiative (Havelock 1973; Lippitt 1973; Tappen 1989).

To address issues arising from conflicting values and beliefs, and to acknowledge the multiple perspectives involved when addressing nursing problems, Hunt (1987) developed an approach with the researcher, practitioner and manager working collaboratively on practice-based change initiatives. Hunt's (1987) approach, which was essentially directed at tackling the issue of resistance to change, epitomizes the collaborative aspects of action research. Resistance to change is, however, not always negative but may be both justified and rational. Resistance is an active process that can stem from factors within the organization, the target group and the change agent often operating in a transactional and reflexive manner. Fear of disorganization and an in-built conservatism can fuel resistance as can a perceived lack of resources and personnel (Schon 1987).

Stability of change is improved if the change spreads to neighbouring systems or subsystems, if there is evidence that it has been positively evaluated in practice and if it was successfully implemented in the face of resistance (Swansburg 1993). Reinforcement and feedback to the target group will improve stability. Also, changes that are visible and have a high profile survive better. Achieving visibility can include publicity such as newsletters, study days and conferences, or whatever seems appropriate to disseminate the news that change has occurred (Swansburg 1993). If the change is to be successfully integrated into the system, the leader needs to establish positive relationships with the target group and should involve the group at each stage in the process. Such collaborative approaches rely heavily on consensus and on a unified appreciation of the need for change (Havelock 1973; Lippitt 1973; Tappen 1989).

Validity in action research

Action research is basically qualitative in orientation and as such it is subjective and recognizes multiple realities. As the method is essentially context specific, action researchers generally do not tend to make claims for generalizability of their findings (Hanson 1994). Action research is therefore not a neutral, value-free process, but is a supporting and questioning initiative that represents a systematic quest for understanding (Titchen 1995). In this approach, the validity criteria include judgements about the relevance, trustworthiness and plausibility of the findings. In keeping with the underlying philosophy, validity is established collaboratively using participant and peer validation to support the results and methods. A decision trail which details the path that the researcher has followed to reach his or her findings can also provide evidence for validation purposes (Titchen 1995).

Reflexivity in the current study

Issues of reflexivity are central to the conduct of action research because the method relies on the researcher, target group and environment all interacting in a dynamic, reflexive manner (Connors 1988; Lamb and Hutlinger 1991; Hanson 1994). A fundamental principle of action research is that the researcher becomes actively involved with those in the action setting, who themselves become active participants in the research effort (Webb 1989). Action research provides a dynamic interaction between research and the organization within which change is being attempted. As a result of its problem-solving, participative style, it has the potential to generate knowledge and to promote positive change in practice. Action research accounts should, however, always highlight any tensions and contradictions within the research field, and should aim to bring the situation under study to life (Meyer 1993).

Over the period of the current study, the researcher–participant relationship altered as a comfortable rapport and shared values developed in relation to caring for the dying patient's relatives. Although such a climate is crucial to the success of a change initiative, it must be acknowledged that this level of reciprocity can have implications for the data that emerge from the study. For the most part, the participating nurses were anxious to be helpful to the researcher. To address issues of potential bias, which such an emotional climate presented, the design of the post workshop evaluation questionnaire and subsequent development of the staff nurses' phase 2 interview schedule were worded specifically to elicit, and encourage, both positive *and* negative responses. The postal questionnaire that evaluated the intervention was also intended to facilitate honest disclosure of the nurses' views and opinions, by offering the nurses the opportunity to comment anonymously on their experiences within the study.

Reflexive influences can also work in a less positive way. In one ward the researcher's regular visits almost invariably seemed to represent an unwelcome interruption. In that ward, the participating nurse was always too harassed to stop for more than a minute (if at all) and the rest of the ward staff were courteous but distant in their manner. Consequently, the researcher always approached that ward with a degree of disquiet predicting, usually rightly, the nature of the reception that she would receive. It provided a graphic illustration of reflexivity. Although a number of efforts were made to support this nurse, the uncomfortable research dynamics that operated were reflected in a low level of commitment to the study by this nurse and consequently by the whole ward team. As a result the standard was never implemented in that ward.

This 'real life' example illustrates that the success of a research initiative and the quality of research data that emerge are variable and affected by a complex web of factors that operate within the research environment.

Ethical issues in action research

Action research relies on the willing cooperation of the target group. The explicit assumption is that action research has a moral base, and that the findings should be advantageous not just to the researcher but should also yield some advantage to the others involved in the study (Waterman 1995). However, change may be potentially threatening and the researcher could well be the catalyst of unwelcome unrest. Meyer (1993) also argues that, as the researcher might be viewed as being in a position of power and coming from another world to which few participants have access, risk of exploitation of participants must be acknowledged and steps must be taken to guard against feelings of abandonment when the researcher disengages.

Conclusion

Change is challenging and exciting; it requires vision and involvement and it represents opportunity (Swansburg 1993). The intervention period in the current study involved the nurses in extensive efforts to implement changes in practice over an extended period of time. During that time, the nurses also developed a range of skills which included developing a standard from research data, negotiating and liaising with a range of personnel, leading and motivating colleagues to change practice, and encouraging them to monitor and evaluate the effectiveness of their care. During this time, the researcher actively sought to provide practical and emotional support and leadership for the staff nurses.

Quality assurance standards provided the mechanism for the ward staff to implement and evaluate changes in their practice. Methot et al. (1992) studied the effects of a standard-setting initiative on staff nurses. The authors suggest that quality assurance standards can empower staff nurses to achieve improvements in the care environment and they can also yield benefits in communication. They conclude that 'there is good evidence that writing and implementing clinical standards can significantly support the processes of planned change' (Methot et al. 1992).

The impact of the intervention on the relatives and the participating nurses is reported in the phase 2 results in Chapters 7 and 8.

Chapter 7
Phase 2 findings: the relatives' accounts

As stated in Chapter 4, a total of 47 interviews were conducted with relatives during the course of the study: 26 in phase 1 and 21 in phase 2. The same instrument, interviewer, approach and analysis strategies were employed in each phase. In acknowledgement of their unique character, each transcript was first analysed as a discrete unit using a line-by-line interpretative approach. Only after this had been completed was cross-referencing of themes across the data set undertaken. A number of major themes and subthemes emerged from the relatives' accounts and these were used for interpreting, organizing and reporting the data.

The phase 2 relatives' data were not in the first instance interpreted with a view to comparison, but were analysed, interpreted and indeed reported in their own right before comparisons were drawn with the phase 1 findings. Dealing with the phase 2 accounts as a completely fresh set of data meant that they could be interpreted in the fullest possible way, rather than merely using them as a vehicle for seeking evidence of change. It was also hoped that this approach would allow new themes to emerge that had not featured in the phase 1 results.

It had been the intention in this chapter to report the findings from the relatives' phase 2 analysis from a wholly non-comparative perspective. Subsequent comparative analysis of the relatives' phase 1 and phase 2 data would then have been reported in Chapter 9, together with data drawn from the standard evaluation processes completed by staff in the study wards. Although the interpretative and reporting processes were undertaken in precisely that way, it was noted that data that emerged from the early parts of the interview were virtually indistinguishable from the phase 1 data. In both relatives' samples, the 'preadmission experiences' were directly comparable in terms of the impact of the diagnosis on the family, the relatives' experiences of care-giving and the emotional conflicts that surrounded the final admission. This finding was not entirely surprising because the study intervention relates specifically to hospital care. Indeed, those differences that did emerge pertained only to the relatives' experiences within the hospital setting.

Furthermore, in the major themes of stress and coping, the phase 2 data were also broadly similar to the phase 1 data in terms of the relatives' reported use of intrapsychic coping strategies such as denial and hope. However, when interpreting these additional data and comparing them with the phase 1 data, deeper insights and understandings were gained into these complex states. Accordingly, to avoid undue repetition when reporting the preadmission experiences and the relatives' responses to the forthcoming death of their loved one, a decision was taken to adapt the reporting of phase 2 findings and this chapter is structured accordingly.

The first section of this chapter offers a summarized account of the phase 2 relatives' 'preadmission experiences'. These data are reported to demonstrate that, where no intervention was applied, no changes were evident. The second section then reports phase 2 data relating to the relatives' stress and coping strategies. Reporting these data should similarly confirm that for both samples the primary source of stress for relatives was their loved one's imminent death. However, it should also enable reporting of new insights gained into the relatives' experiences of stress. The third section reports the remainder of the phase 2 findings and focuses on the relatives' experiences in hospital and their interface with the staff. These data are reported in a way that illustrates similarities to and differences from the phase 1 accounts.

The major themes and subthemes used for reporting the phase 2 data are summarized in Table 7.1.

Phase 2: relatives' 'preadmission experiences'

As stated above, this section offers a summarized version of the phase 2 relatives' data relating to the period before their loved one's final hospital admission. This should confirm that the relatives' experiences were comparable in both phases of the study.

Table 7.1: Themes and subthemes

Preadmission experience	Impact of the diagnosis
	The cancer journey
	Coping with caring
	Crisis intervention
Relatives' stress	Sources of stress
	The experience of stress
Coping and support	Hope, denial and pretence
Distraction and avoidance	Information and coping
	Social support
Hospital as sanctuary	Feelings in conflict
	Privacy and hospitality
	Vigil supported
	Vigil disturbed
Communication	Staff–relative interface
	Caring bonds
	Pathways or walls?
	Information channels
	Supportive interventions
	Experiencing empathy

Theme 1: the preadmission experience

Within this major theme, subthemes include the impact of the cancer diagnosis on the family, relatives' experiences of supporting their loved ones during the course of the illness and providing care at home during the advanced stages of the disease. Also included are the relatives' perspectives about events that led to the final admission. As already stated, only a brief account is given because the phase 2 'preadmission data' are virtually indistinguishable from those reported in the phase 1 findings.

The impact of the diagnosis

The impact of the diagnosis was described in various ways, but seemed to come either as an abrupt shock described in such terms as 'like a 'thunderbolt' or as more of a gradual realization or 'slow dawning' of the gravity of their loved one's illness. Relatives described where, how and by whom the news was delivered. Although sensitive and caring communication was reported by several relatives, around half reported feeling 'desperate' or 'frantic' as they waited for confirmation of the diagnosis. In the exemplar below a man describes hearing his 36-year-old wife's diagnosis.

They expected to find an ovarian cyst or fibroids in the womb . . . [emotional control fragile]. Unfortunately that wasn't the case. When they opened her up they discovered a massive tumour.

Interview no. 2/1

The cancer journey

Fluctuating and intense emotions were described by relatives as their loved one's illness progressed through stages and treatments, causing their own hopes and fears to wax and wane. All were ultimately faced with the realization that the final stages of the illness had been reached and the focus of care must shift to a purely palliative mode. The potential for stress in such unpredictable circumstances is described in the following exemplar.

After seven doses of chemotherapy he was really doing just great. And we went dancing every night . . . . To the sequence dancing. The only thing was he tired easily and we had to maybe leave early. Apart from that he was great. Then he started to feel as though he had the 'flu . . . and he got some antibiotics. But he wasn't really getting any better . . . . He was just so exhausted and worn out . . .

Interview no. 2/15

Coping with caring

Relatives frequently commented on how ill-equipped they had felt to meet their loved one's escalating care needs at home, and they described the stress and the feelings of helplessness that their care-giver role had engendered. Concerns that although at home their loved one was not getting the 'best possible care' were expressed by around half of the relatives, many of whom were themselves elderly. The following exemplar illustrates the nature of the strain that such elderly care-giving relatives can experience.

He needed looking after day and night because he was incontinent so I was up practically the whole night every night changing his pyjamas and changing the bed. I went through an awful lot of linen and the washing machine was always running – as you can imagine. The GP sent his nurses over but it's only recently that they had been coming to help with the bathing. Before that I had to do it all myself.

Interview no. 2/17

Of the 21 relatives interviewed in phase 2 of the study, four reported that the patient had been visited by a district nurse and two of these had also had visits from a cancer nurse specialist. Apart from visits from their GP, most relatives seemed largely to have coped on their own at home. However, it should be noted that around a third of the sample reported that the patient's condition had deteriorated very quickly, thereby hastening the hospital admission. The data suggest that the family's access to community nursing support seemed to rest mainly with the GP and, as it is often nurses who mobilize resources for dying patients and their caring families, lack of access to such support can be significant. The quote below provides an illustrative example of how access to facilities and services can be expedited by a well-informed patient advocate.

> My mum has a friend who is a nurse and she visited regularly. When she saw there was a need for assistance she arranged it. She arranged for someone to give her a special mattress, she got an aid to help her go to the toilet, a seat and so on in her shower, and a good upright armchair for the living room. That was just over the past 3 weeks before she came in to hospital. Prior to that she was able to get out and about.
>
> Interview no. 2/13

The above quote underscores the potential benefits to be gained from access to facilities while the patient is being cared for at home. It also supports findings in the literature that 'well educated, middle-class people' tend to have better access to support and are thus able to employ more efficacious coping strategies (Pearlin and Schooler 1978).

Crisis intervention

The main reasons given for hospital admission were that the patient's symptoms were out of control or that care needs had escalated beyond the coping capacity of the family. The following exemplar is typical of many accounts of events that led to the final hospital admission.

> She couldn't stop being sick. She couldn't drink. She couldn't eat. Everything she took came straight back up. And the pain in her back was . . . [gestures – unbearable].
>
> Interview no. 2/4

This brief report on the phase 2 relatives' preadmission experiences reveals their close similarity to the phase 1 accounts and highlights the emotional vulnerability of the family in the days leading up to the final hospital admission.

Phase 2: relatives' stress and coping strategies

This section of this chapter reports findings in relation to the phase 2 relatives' experience of stress associated with their loved one's illness and their complex intrapsychic coping responses.

Theme 2: relatives' stress

The stress experience

No major differences emerged between phase 1 and phase 2 data in this area. As might have been expected, both groups of relatives reported similar physical and psychological responses to the stress that they were experiencing. In the first quote below a woman describes her responses to her pending loss whereas in the second an elderly man acknowledges that his symptoms are probably arising from his stressed state.

> I've lost about a stone and I'm not eating much. My stomach has been all in knots all the time. The diazepam calms my stomach. I take one before I go to the hospital. Things go through my mind all the time . . . all about the hospital. I've been off work for about six weeks.
>
> Interview no. 2/8

> Stress is there. Many a night I have felt something tight . . . my chest has been *really* tight, and I have had to sit up and do deep breathing. I've got over it right enough but the stress is there.
>
> Interview no. 2/5

The transactional qualities of stress experienced during a loved one's terminal illness are evident in the following quote from a man whose young wife was dying. A powerful image of reciprocal stress is conveyed as the respondent describes his own stress in terms of 'carrying her pain'.

> Where my stress comes from is when Anne is in discomfort. If she's had an easy day or night then I'm going to have an easy day or night. If she's in pain, I get stressed. I'm carrying her pain as well.
>
> Interview no. 2/1

The transactional character of stress evident in the above exemplar is widely supported in the literature (Janes 1992; Folkman 1984). The reflexive nature of the emotional responses within families at this time is also revealed by the elderly man quoted below.

> Mary has highs and lows. If you go away when she's had a high then the next day you still feel elated because things are going well. Then you come in and she's down in the depths of despair again . . . . Highs and lows. [sighs]
>
> Interview no. 2/5

Relatives in both phases reported physical and emotional exhaustion during their loved one's final weeks. The following representative quotes reveal that other demands on relatives often add to the stress experienced by relatives.

> I feel drained. It's just like having jet lag. You are tired all the time and then going home and not sleeping properly. And I'm trying to support the rest of the family. I just tend to keep the tears in.
>
> Interview no. 2/3

> When I leave here I have to go round the wee complex of houses where I stay to give a report on how she is. It's nice but quite frankly it tears you out when you're doing it. But people are interested and you have to let them know. When I come back in I have a glass of whisky and sit for a wee while then I go to bed.
>
> Interview no. 2/5

This all-pervading and unremitting character of the stress that the relatives experience was revealed in both phases of the study. The effects on the wider family are revealed by the young man quoted below. He describes how the combined demands imposed by work, travelling and visiting his dying father in hospital for extended periods meant that he was seeing very little of his wife and two young children.

> I'm not home until 9.30 or 10 o'clock. It does make the day very long and it puts a lot of stress on the family because I'm coming in so late every night.
>
> Interview no. 2/2

A number of sources for the relatives' stress were revealed in the data. Above all their stress came from witnessing the deterioration in their loved one's condition and from the grief associated with their own impending loss. Any evidence of suffering in the patient also resulted in significant stress being experienced by the relative. Relatives who were unable to gain access to staff and to information about their loved one's condition also reported stress. Finally, relatives' stress was exacerbated when basic facilities for their comfort and privacy were lacking.

In both phases of the study, relatives primarily reported stress when the situation felt out of their control and they did not know what to expect next. Data from both samples confirm that relatives appear to need some sort of 'yardstick' to enable them to muster their resources for the difficult days ahead. Well over half of the relatives stated that the information that they needed most of all was to have some idea about 'how long' this very advanced stage of the illness might last. Stress was also reported, again equally in both phases, as a result of difficulties in gaining access to medical staff. Despite nurses' considerable potential to act as advocates in this area, no positive changes emerged from the phase 2 data.

Factors reported in the phase 2 data to reduce the stress experienced by relatives are summarized in Table 7.2.

Although the sources of stress identified in phase 2 do not differ markedly from those in phase 1, the nature and the extent of reported stress were different. Before commenting further on those differences, an analysis of the relatives' coping strategies and their access to sources of support is considered.

Theme 3: coping and support

The literature describes two main coping modes as 'problem focused' and 'emotion focused'. Problem-focused strategies aim to

Table 7.2: Factors that reduce relatives' stress

- Seeing the patient comfortable with symptoms relieved
- Receiving regular update from nurses and doctors
- Carers who know the patient and family
- Patient recognized as 'special' by staff
- Caring manner and friendship of staff
- A private place to retreat to away from the bedside
- Facilities for rest and comfort
- Quiet space and time for the family to be together at the end
- Family members and close friends nearby
- Access to social and pastoral support

remove or modify the stress at source whereas emotion-focused strategies are directed at altering the emotional response to the stress (Wrubel et al. 1981; Folkman 1984). As the impending death of their loved one represents the relatives' primary source of stress, and as this situation was clearly not amenable to change, emotion-focused coping responses predominated in the relatives' data. How these strategies were employed is reported below.

Hope, denial and pretence

Defence mechanisms such as avoidance and denial were reported equally by relatives in phase 1 and in phase 2 of the study. The paradox of denial with insight and the need to sustain some fragments of hope were evident in both sets of data. The concept of hope is complex. Evidence offered in the phase 2 data confirmed the phase 1 findings and enabled deepened insights to be gained in this area. The data appeared to suggest that some measure of hope seemed to be essential, not just to sustain the relatives through their current difficult experience, but also to support and sustain their relationship with their dying loved one. Indeed, for some relatives the prospect of surrendering hope seemed to be almost tantamount to abandonment.

Only five of the phase 2 relatives reported that they had been able to engage in discussion with their loved one about their prognosis. The data hinted that some relatives believed that, if they were openly to acknowledge that death was certain, they might rob their loved one of hope and thus precipitate the parting. This supports findings in the literature that hope, like stress, has reciprocal and transactional qualities in that hopefulness or hopelessness in one person within a relationship has a reflexive effect on the others within that relationship (Scanlon 1989; Perakyla 1991; Herth 1993). The importance of hope, even in the face of the certainty of death, represented a strong and poignant feature in the relatives' data. The following quote from an articulate young businessman underscores the tenacity of this emotion.

> I know that they are not going to aggressively treat the cancer because they have said that right from day one. But I just wonder . . . I still have this wee hope. I suppose everyone has . . .
>
> Interview no. 2/2

Although the man quoted above accepted his father's prognosis on an intellectual level, on an emotional level he still wanted to reject the painful fact. Rejection of the truth, even when it is accepted on a rational level, was evident in a number of the responses. The complex character of hope and denial are revealed in the following exemplar where the woman, although happy to be interviewed, was angry about her mother's deteriorating condition and was having problems accepting the situation.

> They can't take away your hope. I mean you've got to have a wee bit of hope if you've to sit there [at the bedside]. And that's why I can't speak to the doctors . . . because they're trying to destroy it. Where there's life there is hope. I mean I know at the back of my mind that she might not . . . she might not survive . . .
> *Researcher.* But you don't feel quite ready to bring it to the front of your mind?
> No . . . No you can't sit with somebody and be thinking 'I'm going to be burying you shortly'.
>
> Interview no. 2/8

The transactional character of hope and denial parallel closely with 'mutual pretence', a death awareness context first mooted some 30 years ago (Glaser and Strauss 1965). In mutual pretence, although the reality of the forthcoming death is mutually under-stood, all opt to pretend otherwise and accordingly the prospect of the death is not discussed. The current data confirmed that mutual pretence was employed by many families in the study. The complex-ity of these pretence strategies is illustrated in the brief quotes below.

> He [husband] doesn't say a lot . . . He's not telling me a lot. The doctor told me all that's happening but *he'll* not say anything to upset me.
>
> Interview no. 2/15

> I would rather that he didn't know that *we* know until he can say himself. Because I think he's put it out of his mind that he has cancer. He told me once but that was about it . . . that was it.
>
> Interview no. 2/2

The following exemplar underlines the lengths to which pretence can be taken. In it the patient's wife describes the elaborate and collective efforts she and her large family went to as they colluded to protect their dying father from the truth about his condition.

He [husband] would say 'I'm still eating so how am I still losing weight? . . . I would just tell him he was worrying too much. But he wasn't stupid. I think the two of us were kidding each other on . . . Anyway on the Monday he was down to 13 stone [from 15 stone]. And the day he discovered that we all stood on the scales too, one after another, and we all pretended that we were all lighter too. To convince him that the scales were wrong.

Interview no. 2/9

The energy and effort invested in such pretence took its toll, and relatives often reported feeling exhausted and drained by the energy needed to keep up the charade. This is vividly revealed in the following quote from a young woman whose mother is dying. The language used conveys a powerful image of her acting out a part as in a play.

Somehow I feel you get an inner strength as soon as you get to the ward . . . and then you put on your wee smile – and you go in and behave totally naturally. But when you come out you are totally exhausted.

Interview no. 2/8

For many relatives, the prospect of bringing the painful truth out into the open proved just too daunting. The data reveal the inner struggle that can be experienced as relatives seek to move from a mutual pretence situation to an open awareness context. Although examples of open awareness were not common in either phase of the study, a particularly vivid example is provided by the phase 2 relative quoted below. This family all held strong religious convictions which the relative believed had supported them during this time.

Mum told my sister that she knew what was wrong with her and that she knew she didn't have much time left and that was just fine with her. She's just waiting to go and has been for a long time.

Interview no. 2/7

Sometimes awareness took on a more coded form with the prognosis being given tacit acknowledgement without being openly discussed. In the following exemplar, the man had just met with the consultant to be told his father's prognosis and had then gone in to the ward to see his father. The respondent, who described himself and his father as 'men of few words', relayed the following communication:

> My dad said to me 'No so good eh, Jim?' I said 'What Da?' And he said 'Och, you *know* . . . that what the doctor's been telling you.' So I just said 'Aye . . . [deep sigh] Okay Da.' So he knew himself.
>
> Interview no. 2/11

The respondent's use of facial expression and body language as he relayed the above encounter confirmed that father and son had communicated an important message in a way that best suited their own normal patterns of interaction. This supports findings from the literature that 'the very secret of some families' coping success' might lie in their decision not to refer openly to the forthcoming death because to do so would generate more pain than they could bear (Seale 1991; Shea and Kendrick 1995). The stress literature bears this out, confirming that 'purposeful inaction' (Wrubel et al. 1981) or 'inhibition of action' (Lazarus 1985) can also represent rational coping responses.

Distraction and avoidance

The use of distraction as a coping strategy was reported by well over half of the relatives. Two examples are offered below.

> I'm just keeping busy . . . trying to exhaust myself. I go to bed but waken up about 5 o'clock and have to get up. I'm sitting here at 6 in the morning. And I'm not eating. My stomach is churning the whole time.
>
> Interview no. 2/6

> I'm keeping busy all the time. I think it's just that I'm anxious. I keep seeing her face coming into my mind . . . lying in the bed and she's pretty miserable. I think that's just my way of dealing with it.
>
> Interview no. 2/14

Although relatives commonly described 'keeping busy' as a way of handling their stress, the data also revealed a point where the relatives' focus shifted to a more reflective mode. This seemed to correspond with a point where the illness took a downward trajectory, denial was shelved and the bedside vigil commenced.

Although the use of denial and hope, and the allied strategies of distraction and avoidance, represented the predominant coping responses in both phases of the study, other emotion-focused or 'palliative' coping strategies were also reported. The brief quotes below offer examples of the range of strategies described in the phase 2 accounts.

> I tend to do a form of meditation. I switch off and relax. Seven years ago I was ill and the doctor gave me tapes for relaxation. Since November I've used the tapes. It's the only thing that's kept me going. I don't think I could have coped otherwise.
>
> Interview no. 2/3

> He's given me diazepam [GP]. He says I can take up to three a day but I'm only taking one. Unless things really upset me and then I take another one.
>
> Interview no. 2/8

> Well, I'm a great believer in God. I talk to Him and ask 'Dear God give me the strength to get through this'.
>
> Interview no. 2/9

> I tried going back to chapel. I'm a Catholic but a very lapsed one. I feel He's not listening. I have cups of tea. And I cry a lot.
>
> Interview no. 2/8

Social support

The benefits of social support already reported in the literature (Nugent 1988; Wrubel et al. 1981) also emerged from the phase 2 accounts. Relatives who had access to a close social network of family, colleagues and friends reported coping benefits.

> I meet a lot of people and I can talk about it all the time. If I wasn't in the job I was in I might have found it much harder. My family and colleagues support me too.
>
> Interview no. 2/1

> I go to my sisters for support. We all get together if anything goes wrong. We do that in our family if anything goes wrong or goes right. That's just our way of dealing with it.
>
> Interview no. 2/4

Seeking information

Although data from the current study reveal the benefits of information as a coping resource, they also expose some of the complexities of this particular coping strategy. Nevertheless, although information needs were found to fluctuate with the relatives' emotional capacity to confront their situation, when they felt deprived of information relatives reported significant stress. The coping benefits associated with gaining access to information are evident in the quote below.

> If I know what I am dealing with then I can draw in my breath and I can deal with it. But when all of the options are out there . . .and you're balancing them all . . . I find that much more stressful.
>
> Interview no. 2/6

The data reported so far indicate that coping strategies vary considerably, confirming the notion that there is no 'right' way to cope with the imminent death of a loved one. Although the use of hope, denial and pretence is strongly represented in these data, five relatives expressed the wish that it would soon be 'all over' and a few covert references to euthanasia were made.

> This may sound terrible but I hope this is over soon for my mum's sake because it is awful for her. If she knew how she was she would just hate it. [holding back tears]
>
> Interview no. 2/16

> The main feeling I have had this last week is that it is really dragging on. Very much so. I mean my dad is very important to me but I wouldn't have wished this on him.
>
> Interview no. 2/6

For some relatives, despite apparent acceptance of the inevitability of death, a dread of the moment of parting remained and several relatives described their mounting apprehension as they approached the ward. The elderly man quoted below offers a typical example.

> The most stressful time is coming in and not knowing what I am going to find. Even at the moment I come in I can relax a wee bit – because she is still there. Until I come in there is always that fear . . .
>
> Interview no. 2/5

The potential to reduce stress by offering a relaxed greeting, or some simple piece of information as the relative enters the ward, is highlighted in the above quote. The wider potential for supporting relatives of dying patients in hospital forms the focus of the third and final section of this chapter.

Phase 2: relatives' experiences in hospital and their interface with the staff

This section reports relatives' phase 2 data that relate to their experiences of care, communication and support within the hospital environment. In the course of reporting these data, comparisons are drawn by highlighting similarities and differences with the phase 1 relatives' accounts.

Theme 4: hospital as a sanctuary

Data within this major theme relate to the complex and conflicting emotions that many relatives experienced when their dying loved one was admitted to hospital, and the extent to which the ward environment was able to meet the relatives' needs for comfort and privacy during this time. Relatives' emotional responses to the admission are only briefly reported because, like the relatives' 'preadmission experiences', these data bear strong similarities to the phase 1 accounts.

Feelings in conflict

The phase 2 data confirm the phase 1 findings, revealing that, although relief was expressed by almost all of the relatives as they relinquished the role of carer and handed over to the 'experts', around two-thirds of the sample also expressed guilt and regret related to the final admission. Although it was evident that, by the time the patient was admitted to hospital, many relatives had reached the limit of their coping capacity, acute sensitivity to any hint of criticism of their failed attempts to provide care at home was evident. This is illustrated in the following exemplar.

> They [nurses] have suggested that he should have been at home to which I took umbrage. [sounds aggrieved] I mean I had already *tried* . . . and my concern now, and his, is to feel there's something medical around him. That there are people around who know what they are doing.
>
> Interview no. 2/6

Privacy and hospitality

Overall, a more positive picture emerged in relation to this theme. As reported in Chapter 6, the participating staff nurses in all but one of the wards had undertaken to improve the provision of facilities for those relatives who remained in the wards for extended periods, in the days leading up to their loved one's death. The magnitude of the changes that were achieved varied considerably, e.g. in one ward a relatives' room was constructed using the space provided by an alcove in the ward. This newly created room was then furnished and equipped using funds raised by the staff. In another ward, a linen cupboard was re-designated and furnished as a small rest room while in yet another ward the nurses' changing room was also refurbished as a relatives' room.

In several wards, camp beds were purchased to allow relatives to rest as they stayed overnight at their loved one's bedside, and in four wards tea- and coffee-making facilities and crockery were provided for the relatives' use. However, in two of the study wards, initial attempts made by the staff nurses to acquire a private area for relatives met with no success and in these wards no other visible improvements were made in relation to the provision of facilities.

Although the phase 2 accounts confirmed that relatives appreciated the efforts made by staff to ensure their physical comfort, they also commonly referred to the friendly and relaxed atmosphere that they reportedly experienced in the wards. This represents a very strong feature in the phase 2 findings. More than half of the phase 2 relatives (13) made direct reference to the efforts being made by staff to help them to feel relaxed and comfortable in the ward. Only two such comments were offered in the phase 1 accounts.

Vigil supported

Relatives in phase 2 commonly reported that nurses had 'gone out of their way' to accommodate the family. The following exemplar describes measures taken in one ward to accommodate a family with 10 adult 'children' during their father's last days. Although this represents a single incident, it merits reporting because it offers a graphic example of nurses applying the principles of family-centred care.

> They cut off a four-bed room for us because there were so many of the family there . . . to get us away from the corridors. They couldn't have done any more. They gave us the room with the TV and toilet. They gave the two boys [sons]

big chairs [recliners]. They were offered beds but they wanted to be in the room with their dad. They gave us tea and coffee non-stop. Pots of it because we are such a big family . . . . It couldn't have been any better.

Interview no. 2/9

The feelings of comfort that resulted for this large, close family were evident during the interview. It was also clear that this innovative intervention had allowed the family to support each other, and the patient, in the hours leading up to the patient's death. Such data suggest that the climate of acceptance and hospitality experienced by the family represented an important coping resource.

The literature confirms that the bedside vigil is an emotionally demanding experience for the whole family (Hull 1989b; Wros 1993). In particular, Hull (1989b) reports that relatives need to withdraw from the bedside for periods, yet still feel the need to remain in close proximity to the patient. Hull's finding, which emphasizes the value of a private room where relatives can rest and muster their emotional resources, is supported in the current study.

The following exemplar illustrates one woman's response to this facility.

Well, this room is a real bonus. It's a Godsend. I actually prefer coming along here rather than going downstairs to the canteen. Because at this stage sometimes other people just annoy you and coming along here . . . well really it's like a sanctuary. I know there is a TV and magazines but just to come in here to the quietness and just sit. It is just fantastic. If you are sitting all the time (at the bedside) you feel like a zombie and then you're not really there for the other person – it's like a sort of duty thing . . . but if you can get away it is a soothing thing. It even makes dad less demanding.

Interview no. 2/12

As previously stated, staff in some wards had purchased camp beds to improve the comfort of relatives who wished to remain overnight at their loved one's bedside. The phase 2 data reveal that this facility was much appreciated as the elderly woman quoted below confirms.

I have been staying overnight since Wednesday [four nights]. A friend has twice stayed overnight with me. They gave me a bed. That's all you need . . . a wee fold-up bed in beside him. And they brought in a recliner chair for my friend so she could sit there while I got a sleep.

Researcher: Does it help Jim when you're there?

Yes. Oh *yes*. He gets agitated if I'm away.

Interview no. 2/12

This woman went on to explain that both she and her husband were 'more contented' when she was able to stay with him, and yet she knew that if he saw her in need of rest he would insist that she leave. In this situation, the provision of a bed represented a significant coping resource, for both patient and relative. Another relative having expressed appreciation for the comfort offered by a camp bed went on to comment more generally on the hospitality and friendship that she had experienced as she stayed overnight with her dying mother. Her comments are typical of several others.

One of the nurses, a lovely girl, asked me about six times if I wanted tea or coffee. Anything at all. They made up a very comfortable bed . . . a camp bed and it's very comfortable. I just walked out to the corridor any time I wanted and had a cup of tea and toast with them. Just sitting at the desk with the nurses which was very nice.

Interview no. 2/6

Having reported the potential supportive benefits to be gained from improved access to facilities for the relatives' privacy and comfort, evidence is offered below of less positive experiences that were reported in this area. Negative comments about facilities were offered by two relatives and the same relatives described staff as formal and distant. These uncommon findings were derived from one ward in which few positive changes were made during the course of the study and where the staff nurse's reported frustration about lack of facilities ran high. It should, however, be noted that, in two other wards where no substantial improvements in facilities had been achieved, other benefits of the change initiative were evident and relatives' positive experiences of communication and support in those wards were reported. These data will be reported in relation to Theme 5: communication.

Vigil disturbed

The phase 2 data confirmed that relatives' distress during the patient's final days was intensified when the family lacked privacy as they sat with their dying loved one. The exemplars below reveal that, during this emotionally intense period, the relatives' sense of intrusion was exacerbated by noisy reminders that all around them life was going on as normal.

> I wasn't comfortable when he was in a four-bedded room. I just felt he was a bit agitated what with all that was going on around him . . . loud televisions . . . . We were getting to the stage that we couldn't even talk to each other. I felt that the nurses should have asked them to keep the TVs down or else it should be compulsory that they have earphones.
>
> Interview no. 2/15

> When he was moved to a room of his own it was the best thing. He was more comfortable. He was happier and we were more comfortable. We could sit there with privacy. There were children coming into the ward which we felt was disturbing too. Don't misunderstand me I know they need to have their families up to see them. But the way we were feeling we just wanted to be alone.
>
> Interview no. 2/6

The above quotes suggest that a point in the journey is reached when the family need to be together in quietness and privacy. The data offered revealing insight into the relatives' needs at this stage. It appears that as distraction and avoidance behaviour are put aside the relatives' primary needs are to be quiet and reflective when at the bedside, and they also need to be able to retire to a quiet, private area when taking a break from the bedside vigil. These findings are supported in the literature. Davies (1990) describes this point in the terminal illness as 'the transition of fading away', whereas Perakyla (1991) refers to it as the point where 'hope is dismantled so that death can be faced'.

Nurses can support relatives during this emotionally intense period if they remain alert and sensitive to the subtle shifts that occur in the family's interactions and take steps to ensure that a quiet area is provided where the patient and family can be together. Nurses should also take steps to ensure the comfort of relatives both at the bedside and in a rest area within the ward.

Discomforts experienced by relatives who stayed overnight in wards that lacked facilities for their comfort were described by two respondents. In the exemplar below, the experiences of a woman called back from the USA to be with her dying father are described. At the time of the interview this family were maintaining a round-the-clock vigil in the ward with screens around the bed.

> No you're not comfortable. I put two of these seats together with a stool in between and tried to lie down. My legs and feet were swelling up because I had sat upright all the time. These chairs are fairly comfortable to sit on for a short time, but when you are sitting all night long it's difficult. The staff are fine as regards tea and toast. They couldn't do enough for you. But you're not comfortable in the sense that you could relax. I know it's difficult with lack of resources in the hospital but I feel in a case like this where time is so short a single room would be just ideal . . . .
>
> Interview no. 2/3

The relatives' reported experiences suggest that access to amenities such as a single room in the days leading up to the patient's death, if indeed this is what the patient and family wish, and to a private area for periods of rest away from the bedside, can represent important coping resources during a time of intense stress for the family.

Other major sources of support for the dying patient's family focus on aspects of communication.

Theme 5: communication

Data reported within this theme focus on mechanisms for establishing contact between relatives and staff, relationships between staff and the dying patient's family, and a range of complex processes that relate to relatives' information needs.

The staff–relative interface

The most distinguishing feature of the phase 2 relatives' data was the frequency of comment about the climate of friendship and warmth that relatives reportedly experienced in the wards. The data strongly indicate that improvements had occurred in the quality of the relationships between dying patients' relatives and nurses in most of the study wards. The following exemplars confirm that this more relaxed ward climate was appreciated by the relatives.

They are talking to me. Asking how my mum is and asking how I am. I would say over the past few days I feel that the nurses are concentrating more on me . . . well maybe not more on me but just as much on me, and my well-being, as caring for my mother.

Interview no. 2/13

They are very caring. Very compassionate. I think they really *do* care . . . . Taking you in to talk to you and taking time with you. And you can *feel* . . . you feel that they really mean it. That they're being sincere.

Interview no. 2/12

Caring bonds

The data also suggested that relatives derived comfort from seeing an emotional bond develop between the nurses and their dying loved one. Relatives reported that they felt reassured to know that the nurses recognized their loved one as 'special' and would care for, and care *about*, them if the relatives had to leave the ward. The support that relatives derived from these caring bonds is clearly demonstrated in the following quotes.

Some nurses put in that wee bit extra. They treat her as a little friend. They'll come up and chat to her and say 'cheerio' before they go home and then come right up to her when they come on duty again.

Interview no. 2/8

It's very comforting to me just knowing that they are there and not just for their medical expertise but their comfort as well. They are so friendly towards my mum and to the whole family. That it is really excellent. It has made a big difference.

Interview no. 2/13

I think maybe it's that they're more like a friend than a nurse. And they are so friendly in the things that they say to him [husband]. It's not as though it's just a job, it's because they want to be a *friend*. To be a bit more.

Interview no. 2/6

Although such indications of liking and respect for the patient were experienced as supportive and comforting, any perceived lack of respect for their loved one understandably generated distress. Although only two such examples emerged from the phase 2 analysis, both are reported to acknowledge the hurt experienced when relatives believe their loved one to be denied due respect.

The doctors did their rounds and never came near him. I just felt that they were treating him as a lost cause. I wouldn't like to be lying there and realize that. Then the nurse was taking his blood pressure and another nurse said 'No don't do that just come back.' I'm not being critical but it's just like he's a lost cause . . . . That really stuck in my throat. They didn't come over even to take a pulse. Anything. Just to make him feel he was still worth having a look at.

Interview no. 2/3

Yesterday a doctor came to see my mum just as I arrived at the bed and he said 'Could you give me a few seconds?' I said 'sure' and went outside. He pulled the screens round and as I walked to the door I heard him say 'Well, I don't think there's anything more can be done here.' I thought 'He's going to say something else' but the next thing screens were pulled back and he walked out. I thought 'No. Surely I haven't heard this'.

Interview no. 2/14

The data suggest that, when the emotional climate in the ward was warm, and the relationships that operated among staff, patients and relatives were positive, this was experienced as supportive by the relatives. The extent to which the ward climate might influence other key aspects of communication, such as the strategies that relatives adopt to make contact with staff and their access to information about their loved one's condition and care, are reported below.

Pathways or walls?

The phase 1 findings, from both relatives and nurses, revealed that it was unusual for nurses to initiate contact with the relatives. Indeed the onus generally lay with the relatives to make the approach. The data also revealed that nurses' hesitancy about making contact was mainly because they did not know what to say, or were unsure about how to handle the relatives' questions. The relatives' phase 1 data confirmed that they also felt hesitant about approaching staff, believing that nurses were too busy to be disturbed. Every relative in phase 1 expressed concern that by approaching staff they might be seen as a nuisance.

In contrast, the phase 2 data offered evidence that in most of the study wards staff now regularly make the initial approach to relatives. Relatives reported deriving support from the friendly informality with which the staff–relative contact was now being established. The comments below offer typical examples in this area.

Most definitely the nurses approach me. I haven't had to go and seek out a nurse out at all. They obviously sense your need.

Interview no. 2/6

The nurses have approached me but I think they've done it so diplomatically that it looks as if it was a little chat. I think it's a good idea if staff approach the relative first without making it sound as if it was some deadly serious information. More as if they're just in the habit of having a chat.

Interview no. 2/10

When we came in this time Staff Nurse S . . . immediately came up to us and said who she was and that she would be looking after Mary.

Interview no. 2/5

One young man, whose father was now close to death, reflected on and described his experience of communication which was sensitive to his changing needs as he adjusted to his father's prognosis.

I was still finding it very difficult to come to terms with what was happening and I knew that the sister was trying to tell me, to prepare me for it. At times I didn't want to see her but looking back it was my failure to accept the situation. Looking back it really was the right thing. The way she handled it was almost like a textbook – it just started off as a gentle 'hello' building up to having a conversation about him.

Interview no. 2/2

Overall the phase 2 data offered evidence that in the study wards the nurses now adopted a more relaxed approach with relatives and regularly engaged them in conversation. These findings differ from those in phase 1 where it was revealed to be uncommon for nurses to initiate contact with relatives or for relatives to have a 'conversation' with staff. The phase 1 finding that the onus for initiating contact usually rested with the family has also been confirmed in the literature (Lugton 1987; Hull 1989b; Dunlop and Hockley 1990). Two relatives in phase 2 reported lack of contact with nurses. One was a distressed, angry woman who was having difficulty accepting her mother's fatal prognosis. A quote from this woman is provided because it offers insight into the feelings of isolation (and desolation) that can result when relatives lack contact with the staff.

I'm not even just talking about facilities . . . [weeping quietly] But just to have a
nurse greet you . . . not necessarily as a long lost friend . . . but just so that if you
have any questions you can go to her. If they could just come over and say a wee
word . . . just let you know if he's had a bad night or whatever. That way you
would know. I mean it's a job to them but it's family to me. That way you would
see there was a wee bit of care there . . . a wee bit of attention.

Interview no. 2/16

Such data suggest that relatives' stress levels increase and their
level of concern for their dying loved one can escalate when staff
adopt a distant manner towards the family. The relative quoted
above experienced unmet needs for information, yet clearly felt
constrained about seeking this out in a climate that she judged to be
unsupportive. This situation should, however, be set fully and fairly
in context. The father of the woman quoted above was being
temporarily cared for in another ward while the study ward closed
for upgrading and for construction of a relatives' room. Although
not offering a true representation of phase 2 data in the sense that
the location and some of the ward staff had changed, the quote is
included for the revealing insights that it offers.

Information channels

Relatives in both phases of the study had quite definite ideas about
what nurses could tell them and what they believed should correctly
come from a doctor. Although information about treatment and
prognosis was seen to be firmly in the doctors' domain, relatives
defined 'nurse information' as 'an update on the patient's day-to-day
general condition and overall comfort'. Commonly expressed views
in this regard are exemplified in the quote below.

Staff nurses are only allowed to tell you so much. They can't go above a doctor.
They can't tell you certain things. I'm wise enough to know that. Apart from
that anything I've asked them they were quite helpful.

Interview no. 2/9

In contrast with the phase 1 findings, very few problems were
reported in phase 2 in obtaining information from nursing staff.
However, a third of the relatives reported difficulties in getting information from doctors. The stress that unmet needs for information
engenders is illustrated in the following exemplars.

> When I arrived here [from Canada] on the Monday I wanted so much to talk to
> the doctor. Not so much the nurses. I wanted to talk to the doctor. I was told by
> the nurses that tests were going on. It took me until the following Monday to get
> an appointment.
>
> Interview no. 2/7

> When we eventually saw Dr D he was charming. He answered all our questions
> and then he said 'You know you could have got me here in the ward any morn-
> ing'. And we thought, 'Well why has it taken us *weeks* to get to speak to you?' It's
> not right. Nurses should put themselves in our position. We wanted to know
> what was happening . . . what the prognosis was. We just wanted to know.
>
> Interview no. 2/6

The relative quoted above clearly believed that nurses should
intervene to expedite the family's access to medical staff. The
phase 2 results offer no firm evidence that nurses have taken any
additional initiatives in this regard. The following quote confirms
that relatives feel hesitant about making a formal request to see
medical staff for information, confirming that the potential exists
for nurses to act in an advocacy role on behalf of the family in this
regard.

> I feel uncomfortable about going and asking the doctors because I know they are
> awful busy. If there's not any change you feel a bit silly having to go and ask. I
> would feel happier if they [doctors] made the first move . . . because it is a very
> difficult time. You feel that you don't want to ask. Although you want to know –
> somehow you don't want to ask . . . . You want the information given voluntarily.
>
> Interview no. 2/13

Confirming the potential for nurses to function as relatives' advocates, the final exemplar in this section reveals an elderly man's difficulties with the terminology used during his discussions with the
medical staff.

> Although they [medical staff] are very caring it's just that sometimes they have a
> manner that's a wee bit above you. And you have to ask about things . . . It's
> really like a different language.
>
> Interview no. 2/5

It has been confirmed in both phases of this study that regular
access to information represents an important coping resource for
relatives and that, when they feel deprived of information, relatives

experience stress. This finding is also widely supported in the literature (Weisman 1979; Wrubel et al. 1981; Hull 1989b, 1992).

The phase 2 data have revealed a wide range of nursing interventions that relatives found supportive. Some of these have been reported elsewhere in this chapter and so are only briefly summarized below.

Supportive interventions

The high value that relatives placed on social support provided by nursing staff in the study wards was established earlier in this chapter. Most relatives in phase 2 of the study described the ward climate and the manner and attitude of the nursing staff as comforting and supportive. Relatives' feelings of distress were primarily alleviated by nursing activities specifically directed at keeping the patient comfortable and free from distressing symptoms. Next in the relatives' priority was to receive regular and detailed information about the patient's condition and care and in particular to get regular access to the medical staff.

The phase 2 data reveal that relatives derived comfort from dealing with nurses who were known to the family and who also seemed to know and *like* the patient. The data revealed that warm, friendly staff who took time to talk to the relatives, and to listen to them, were frequently reported as important sources of support. The closer and more relaxed relationships reported between nurses and relatives were a marked feature in the phase 2 accounts. Findings relating to ward facilities were also strikingly different from the phase 1 data. With few exceptions, relatives seemed generally to feel more at ease in the ward and they appreciated the provisions that were being made in many of the wards for their privacy and comfort. Frequent reference was made to the friendship that staff in many wards now extended to the relatives.

Relatives' final comments

The opportunity to make further comment was offered at several stages in the interview and at the end of each interview. Most of the relatives accepted this invitation. Although the nature of their comments varied, most were highly complimentary of nursing staff. These comments highlighted the nurses' considerable potential for alleviating stress and for providing support for people as they face the impending loss of a loved one.

During this final part of the interview unmet needs were also expressed by a few relatives. These mainly related to the relatives' needs for improved access to medical staff and to 'medical' information about their loved one's condition and care. Two relatives referred to the discomforts they had experienced as a result of a lack of basic facilities for their comfort and privacy.

The potential for relatives' anxiety to be increased when they perceive a lack of support and understanding from staff is revealed in the following exemplar.

> Most of the nurses are understanding but I think you have to be in this situation yourself before you realize what you need.
> *Researcher*: You are in the situation now, Carol. You can help us to know.
> Well, I don't want sympathy because that just upsets you. I think just a little understanding about John having to go out of hospital [Carol terrified that John will be discharged] and about us not getting to see a doctor when we really needed to. A lot of people do want to know. I know it might be their patient . . . but it's still *our* dear one.
>
> Interview no. 2/6

The relatives' phase 2 data confirm that relatives recognize and appreciate the extra effort and commitment that many nurses display. When nurses reduce the emotional distance and connect with the family, a sense of empathy is conveyed from which relatives derive considerable support. Although the exemplar below represents a particularly lucid and strong example, similar sentiments were expressed by several other relatives.

Experiencing empathy

> The nurses have to realize that in dealing with relatives in my situation it's just different from a normal patient's visitors. You have got to have that little bit extra. Possibly some of the nurses won't have that little bit extra to give. But I've discovered some of these nurses *do* have it.
>
> *Researcher*: How does that 'little bit extra' help?
>
> It just reassures me that Peter is going to be all right. That they've got his interest at heart – and *mine*. It makes me feel better when I can feel that contact between them and I think 'she's a lovely girl – she knows . . . she *feels*'.
>
> Interview no. 2/6

Chapter 8
Phase 2 findings: the staff nurses' accounts

As stated in Chapter 4, 15 staff nurses were interviewed during phase 2 of the study. These interviews differed from the phase 1 interviews in several ways. Although the same nurses were interviewed, a shorter, more focused interview approach was adopted in phase 2 and the instrument also differed in that it was designed to revisit issues that were explored in the nurses' phase 1 interviews, and to address issues and concerns raised during the course of the intervention.

The researcher–participant relationship had also changed because, by then, we had known each other for some 18 months and were on friendly informal terms. Issues of reflexivity inherent in such an extended participant–researcher relationship within a collaborative endeavour are discussed in Chapter 4 and are also addressed in Chapter 6, which describes the intervention.

During the course of the phase 2 interviews, the nurses spontaneously sought to contextualize their current perceptions by reflecting back on their feelings and experiences at different stages in the process in which they had become involved. Consequently the phase 2 data emerged already cast in a comparative mould and could not be analysed in isolation from the phase 1 data. As had occurred in phase 1, the phase 2 interviews were audio-taped and transcribed into the textual analysis software package (Padilla 1993).

From the analysis processes a number of major themes and subthemes emerged and these formed the framework for interpreting and reporting the data. These are summarized in Table 8.1.

Table 8.1: Major themes and subthemes

Themes	Subthemes
Stress and coping	Sources of stress
	Coping responses
	Peer support
	Reciprocal support
	Increased comfort
Facilities for families	'The room' as a symbol
	Impact on communication
	Impact on coping
Interprofessional issues	The boundaries
	Breaking the mould
	Collaborative approach
Participants' perspective	Effects on facilitators
	Impact of the data
	Impact of the workshop
	Impact on care
	Support and solidarity
	Frustrations along the way

Thematic analysis

Stress and coping

Aspects of stress and coping were omnipresent and interwoven throughout the data. Themes reported in this category include sources of stress for nurses, the coping strategies that nurses employed, the nurses' access to support and the degree of comfort that they currently experience with this aspect of their role.

Sources of stress

Stress caused by trying to respond sensitively to the needs of the dying patient and family while working in an acute hospital ward was reported by virtually every nurse in phase 1 of the study, whereas this was raised as a concern by only three nurses in phase 2. The following exemplars reveal that, while the wards do not seem less busy, and staffing levels are reported as the same, or in some cases worse than when the phase 1 interviews were conducted, the nurses' appraisal of the situation as stressful and their ways of responding to the demands that they face appear to have altered.

I find the whole ward so bad at the moment. It stinks at the moment. They are cutting staff numbers back and you are frantic all the time. If people need you to sit with them then other things are left until later.

Interview no. 8

We need more staff and more time to spend with people because it's stressful trying to talk to someone while at the back of your mind are all the other things you have to do. But I feel I *am* finding it all less stressful. I find I can now say 'well that can just wait'.

Interview no. 4

These data suggest that a shift may have occurred in the priority now being afforded to the dying patient's family and that the nurses' perceptions of the situation may have changed. Although the pressures of competing demands have not changed, it seems that now 'other things', and not the distressed family, have to wait. However, although there was evidence in the phase 2 data to suggest that most nurses now appraised this aspect of care as less threatening than before, some still reported feelings of helplessness in the face of the relatives' suffering. The nurses' feelings in this area are typified in the following quotes.

It's the relatives you are hurting more for. As long as the patients are comfortable and pain free the hardest part is the relatives. You can just imagine what they are going through.

Interview no. 10

You can't really ease their suffering and you know what the outcome is going to be. That's what makes it feel so bad. You feel sort of helpless in a way.

Interview no. 2

Stress engendered by having to deal with relatives' emotional responses, and particularly their anger, was reported by most of the nurses in their phase 1 interviews, but only two such reports were made in phase 2. One of these is included here because it offers such a graphic illustration of the difficulties that nurses can experience when dealing with displaced anger. The exemplar also confirms that, even in the face of substantial improvements in care and facilities, there can still be situations that defy comfort.

If someone is upset you can give them comfort and a hug but if someone is angry I still find that hard. You know you are trying your hardest but they'll still pick on something which to us seems trivial and unimportant but to them is a big issue. If they are angry there's nothing you can do. You can try to stay calm to defuse the situation but if that's the stage they're going through . . . well I do still find that hard.

Interview no. 5

Although the nurse quoted above displays considerable insight into the relatives' plight, the stress that can result from such angry encounters is nevertheless evident. Even when it is acknowledged that the relatives' responses probably result from their grief and distress, it is understandable that nurses might feel distressed when such emotions are directed at them.

Overall, however, an easing of tensions between nurses and relatives is suggested in the phase 2 data. This observation was supported by fewer reports of encounters with angry relatives and by the complete absence of the conflict-laden language, evidenced by war metaphors, which had been a notable feature in the nurses' phase 1 data, especially within the context of the nurse–relative communication.

Nurses' self-reported levels of stress had also changed during the course of the study. When presented with a 4-point Likert scale, all but one respondent in phase 1 of the study rated this aspect of care as being either 'fairly stressful' or 'very stressful', with more than half opting for 'very stressful'. One chose 'slightly stressful' and no one opted for 'not stressful'. In the phase 2 responses the nurses' self-ratings of stress were almost equally divided between 'slightly stressful' and 'fairly stressful'. One (as compared with eight in phase 1) judged this aspect of care to be 'very stressful'.

However, although all but two nurses claimed in their phase 2 interviews that the levels of stress that they experienced when providing support for the dying patient's relatives had now reduced, such comments often contained caveats such as 'of course, it can't ever be stress free' or 'if you don't feel any stress at all then you're not doing it right'. Acknowledgement that the very nature of this difficult situation defies comfort is suggested in the following exemplar.

I probably still take an awful lot of it home with me [stress] and I can go home feeling quite sad about some of the cases that we nurse. I don't think that will ever leave me and I don't know if I would ever want it to.

Interview no. 3

Although the source of the nurses' stress had not altered, in that they still had to deliver care within an emotionally charged situation, the phase 2 data revealed that the nurses' perceptions of 'feeling stressed' had changed. These altered perceptions of stress might be attributable to changes in the nurses' coping responses and their judgements about the support currently available to them.

Coping responses

It was confirmed in Chapter 3 that problem-focused and emotion-focused coping strategies tend to be used synchronously in the management of stress, although the dominance of one approach over the other will vary with the stressful situation's potential for amelioration (Pearlin and Schooler 1978).

The nurses' phase 1 data revealed a preponderance of emotion-focused or 'palliative' coping strategies and, although similar coping measures were reported in phase 2, the nature and extent of their use differed, e.g. although the phase 1 data reveal liberal use of avoidance and distancing behaviour, such evidence was almost entirely absent in the phase 2 accounts. Moreover, as the following exemplar illustrates, the nurses' judgements about their own coping resources also appear to have changed.

> The relatives still take up an awful lot of your time. Personally, since the study started I've found I've been able to jiggle my time about better so that I don't feel that panic and that rush when I speak to people. That's something I've learnt in the past two years. But they do need a lot of your time and attention. But it's a different priority now. I remember during the workshop other nurses were saying that they looked at their watches and thought 'Oh God, I'm running out of time and I've still got my drug round to do.' I don't do that anymore. I speak to people first.
>
> Interview no. 3

Changes were evident in the range and extent to which palliative coping measures were reportedly used. The phase 2 data reveal an increase (from two to seven respondents) in the use of self-nurturing strategies such as aromatherapy, exercise and/or relaxation as part of the nurses' coping repertoire. Strategies such as 'ranting and raving' or 'crying at home', reported by almost a third of the nurses in phase 1, were much less in evidence in the phase 2 data. The following quotes illustrate some of the coping strategies reported in the nurses' phase 2 data.

> I go out and have a wee drink sometimes if I'm really stressed. And getting home where there's no noise I find that's really good.
>
> Interview no. 2

> I do a lot more aerobics than I used to. I find that's really good. And just going home and relaxing . . . getting away from it.
>
> Interview no. 11

> I used to smoke but I've stopped now so I go to the gym now. I spend about an hour and a half in the gym, swimming pool and Jacuzzi and I just chill out. I feel a *lot* healthier now.
>
> Interview no. 12

> I find now when I've had a really bad early shift I go and swim and this is something that I picked up from the workshop . . . . It's very worthwhile.
>
> Interview no. 3

> My closest friend is a nurse. It's great to have her because she knows exactly what I'm on about and vice versa. Someone to listen so that we can get it off our chests. I think I also cope with it now by showing my feelings. You have to let go and not bottle things up.
>
> Interview no. 10

The ability to compartmentalize concerns associated with professional and private life represented one nurse's reported strategy. The exemplar below highlights an interesting, if singular, approach to managing work-related stress.

> When I leave the ward I try to leave all my worries and troubles behind and pick them up when I come back in the door. Once I get changed I think of what I'm doing tonight or what's happening . . . . It's a conscious switch.
>
> Interview no. 6

It was revealed in Chapter 3 that a history of past coping success can exert a positive influence on an individual's evaluations of their ability to meet new challenges. This belief in one's own capacity to cope with stress has been described in the literature as a 'sense of coherence' (Strumpfer 1990; Larsson et al. 1994). The nurses' data indicate that past experiences of stress, in both their personal and professional lives, can influence the nurses' evaluations of their ability to cope with the stress involved in caring for dying patients and their families. In the phase 2 accounts, frequent reference was made to the increased confidence and sense of mastery that had resulted when the nurses felt that they had successfully met these challenges when dealing with relatives of dying patients in their wards. Several nurses also reported that, as a result of their enhanced insight into relatives' concerns and needs, and their own recent more positive experiences of providing this type of care, their subjective feelings of feeling stressed were reducing.

> The feedback from the relatives' interviews helped a lot. Because now you know that even though you think you are just sitting there and can't offer any answers . . . you know now that just *being there* has made a difference.
>
> Interview no. 8

The following quote offers a particularly poignant example of a nurse whose 'sense of coherence' and mastery (Strumpfer 1990) resulted from having faced a major coping challenge in her past private life.

> My dad died in a car crash when I was thirteen. That was the most horrific thing that could ever happen. It was awful at the time but just somehow you get inner strength and you just have to get on with it. I always go back to that. If I could cope with that then I can cope with anything. That's the worst thing to ever happen to me. Nothing could ever equal that.
>
> Interview no. 10

The nurse quoted above is employing the strategy of cognitive reformulation which involves manipulating perceptions of situations in an effort to reduce their stressful impact (Folkman 1984). By placing the catastrophic event of her father's death on a scale of stressors, other potentially stressful situations, such as coping with relatives of dying patients, pose a relatively lesser threat.

Peer support

The phase 2 data indicate that, in many of the study wards, staff now regularly engage in discussion about issues that surround caring for dying patients and in particular about supporting the family.

Ventilating anxieties in this way appears to have had the effect of rendering the situation less stressful and increasing the nurses' comfort when dealing with the dying patient's relatives. The data seemed to suggest that, within the ward teams, a sense of solidarity in the face of a common challenge was emerging.

> We are now more open with each other. They [ward nurses] can all see that it's not something that they have to cope with by themselves . . . and that if at times they don't cope then that's not a failure. It's not seen now that you are any less a nurse or any less a person.
>
> Interview no. 1

> I find I can approach relatives more easily now. And I think it's just the feeling that you are not the only one. We are all feeling more or less the same way. It's nice to know you are not alone.
>
> Interview no. 14

Peer support within the ward team seems to enable a more positive reappraisal to be made of the threat that this aspect of care presents, and helped reaffirm the nurses' confidence in their ability to cope with the demands of the situation. The problem-solving elements of staff discussions appeared to facilitate reflection on and analysis of current practice, thus enabling proposed changes in practice to be discussed and agreed. Engaging in positive action in this way represents an important coping strategy because the feelings of empowerment that can be generated have the potential to lessen psychological and physical distress. These commonly expressed views in the phase 2 interviews are exemplified in the quote below.

> I think in our ward it's the fact that we've actually sat down and discussed family support. We talked about it and realized that a lot of us were just scared of what we were going to be asked. We've made sure we all realize what we are able to tell relatives and when we can pass things on.
>
> Interview no. 7

Reciprocal support

When friendly informal relationships developed between nurses and relatives this was perceived as mutually supportive, thus underscoring the transactional and reciprocal characteristics of stress and coping discussed in Chapter 3 (Wrubel et al. 1981; Folkman 1984). The phase 2 data reveal that many nurses had previously held unrealistic expectations of themselves and that, in the light of insights that they had gained from the phase 1 data, they could now recognize that providing support for the dying patient's family was within their coping capacity. The following exemplar illustrates the reflexive and dynamic character of coping and the effects that such a climate of reciprocity can have on nurses' judgements about the threat that this aspect of their practice presents.

> Over the months a lot of the staff are finding it easier to approach relatives. You try to build up relationships so the relatives feel more at ease approaching you. In turn we all feel better about approaching them.
>
> Interview no. 10

The phase 2 data reveal reports of reciprocal benefits emerging in most wards from the warmer relationships that had been established between nurses and relatives. The very representative quote offered below highlights the potential for reciprocal support that such relationships can yield.

> I would say it's fairly stressful at times but in a way I feel I'm getting more back from relatives. You feel you are doing a good job now. Before there were times when I felt I just wasn't doing it properly and I felt really uptight because of that. Now I feel that I'm meeting more of the relatives' needs and, because I feel that, I'm not as stressed.
>
> Interview no. 15

Increased comfort

The above quote reveals the stress that nurses experience when they feel dissatisfied with the care that they deliver, and it also highlights the resulting reduction in stress when they are able to feel satisfied with their practice. This supports evidence from the literature that, when nurses are frustrated in their attempts to deliver care that is congruent with their own personal values, they can become emotionally exhausted, disillusioned and 'burned out' (Oberle and Davies 1993). The phase 2 data appear to support the view that, when caring relationships are established with the dying patient's relatives, the nurses' stress is reduced and they report increased comfort in their role. Evidence of the nurses' increased comfort was further supported by the absence of conflict-laden language (war metaphors) which had featured in the phase 1 accounts.

> It has changed for me. I try to make a point now of going in when the relatives arrive and explaining what has been happening and then I say 'if you want to speak to me later just come and find me'. I try to do that now, even in cases where it's difficult. Before I might have tried to avoid talking to them.
>
> Interview no. 8

> I'm a lot more comfortable than I was before we started this study. A *lot* more. I feel more secure in myself now. Better equipped to deal with it. I don't feel alone anymore. I feel there are others that know too . . . so you don't feel isolated. It's a team.
>
> Interview no. 13

In their capacity as facilitators, the participating staff nurses were responsible for encouraging participation from their colleagues in the ward team. Around half of the phase 2 accounts contained references to the ward colleagues' commitment to the initiative. The following quotes are typical of many others.

> Our main concern before was just with the patient, and the relatives came second. But now, myself and the others in the ward are equally caring and concerned about patients and relatives.
>
> Interview no. 14

> We are all more aware of relatives now. I feel that I can approach them more easily now. The other staff in the ward are aware of the study and the standard is up and running. They have really been quite involved.
>
> Interview no. 15

The phase 2 data indicate that to varying degrees in most of the nursing teams changes in awareness of relatives' needs and alterations in attitudes and practices had occurred. The extent to which the staff nurse facilitators and their teams were able to achieve improvements in facilities for the dying patient's family is considered below.

Facilities for families

A common concern for both nurses and relatives in the phase 1 data related to lack of facilities and accommodation for families of dying patients. During the intervention the nurses identified the need to improve this aspect of care, and in all but two of the wards efforts were made to implement changes in this area.

The 'room' as a symbol

The importance of physical factors such as accommodation and facilities should not be underestimated. Indeed the data from this study suggest that the provision of a private room for relatives holds almost symbolic importance to nurses. This view is wholly understandable when we stop to consider that, in the course of dealing with the dying patient's family, nurses frequently find themselves in stressful and emotionally charged encounters where their own coping resources are severely challenged. In such circumstances, to be able to offer something tangible can assume major significance. Providing a private sensitive area where relatives can rest and have private discussions with staff seemed to confirm the relatives' legitimate place in the plan of care. Indeed, the relatives' room appeared to offer the nurses a visible means of conveying their commitment to family support.

Some of the nurses' successes and frustrations as they strove to improve ward facilities for relatives are described using illustrative exemplars.

> I feel that in setting up the relatives' room we've done well. It's been nice to have this for people to come to. It's somewhere for them to come and be away if they need a break from their relatives. It's a nice cosy room. I wish it was bigger and had better facilities but it's getting there.
>
> Interview no. 3

> Although we have always had a relatives' room, it is much more comfortable now and we have managed to get tea- and coffee-making facilities, and comfortable, reclining chairs that they can sleep in rather than just those wee chairs from around the ward.
>
> Interview no. 4

Impact on communication

Such a facility also affords privacy to both the relative and nurse during what might well be emotionally intense encounters. The 'feel good' factor that achieving this facility provides for nurses should, therefore, not be underestimated or trivialized. Anything that increases physical and emotional comfort and reduces tension between nurses and relatives might have the potential to improve communication, enhance coping and reduce stress.

The following exemplars, both from nurses who work in the same ward, describe their efforts to provide accommodation for relatives by having a room constructed from an alcove in the ward corridor. Having obtained the necessary permission from their nurse manager to secure this major structural change in the ward, these young nurses negotiated with a range of personnel. The lengths they went to, and the frustrations they experienced, are vividly revealed below.

> We have spoken to the estates manager who has assured us that the room will definitely be built when the ward closes for redecoration. We've been in touch with the WRVS with regard to helping to furnish it. And there's ward funds – we've just been left money from a lady who died – so we're hoping to buy a tea set for the room.
>
> Interview no. 10

> I am a lot more positive about it now. I think that, when you spoke to me before [first interview], I was saying 'well what can we do?' I felt I was banging my head off a brick wall. There were no facilities for the relatives. But now at least we have something concrete to go on so there is a little bit more hope than there was a year or so ago.
>
> Interview no. 12

The following quote, from a nurse in another ward where substantial changes in the provision of facilities were made, confirms that a critical factor in the nurses' level of commitment to change and their subsequent success in achieving it was the support and encouragement that were provided by their nurse manager.

> Our nurse manager has been very supportive. She found out about our study when it changed to the NHS Trust and Directorate and she really was all for it.
>
> Interview no. 3

In another ward in the same hospital, the nurses had similarly hoped to have changes made to create a private area for relatives. However, these nurses were unable to carry their plan through because, they claim, they lacked the necessary support from their nurse manager. The nurses' perceptions about their lack of success at effecting changes in this area had far-reaching consequences because it affected their motivation to improve other aspects of care. The level of frustration this engendered is revealed in the following quote.

> There's just nowhere for relatives at the moment. A Parker Knoll at the side of the bed is all right – but it's not what you would want is it? I just don't think people have realized the necessity for privacy. But when you see relatives and friends in corridors weeping their eyes out . . . . *That's just not on* . . . That's my main frustration.
>
> Interview no. 13

Impact on coping

The importance of having an appropriate setting within which to communicate with the dying patient's family has emerged from this theme. The complex interrelationships that exist between the provision of suitable accommodation for relatives and the quality of communication that takes place between staff and relatives is evident in the following exemplar.

> At the start of the study I think I said that it is quite difficult to know what to say to the relatives. But now with the room being here, it does help. You can actually sit down and talk to the family.
>
> Interview no. 9

These data also suggest that the level of the nurses' and relatives' stress can be moderated and their coping efforts enhanced by the provision of appropriate facilities for relatives who have to spend extended periods of time in the wards. The data also suggest that interactions between nurses and relatives are influenced by a range of interrelated factors which operate within the health-care team. Some aspects of communications within the interprofessional team are considered below.

Interprofessional issues

Data reported within this theme indicate that, although in most wards communication between medical and nursing staff remains to some degree problematic, in three of the study wards there is now clear evidence of dialogue and collaboration between the professions. Overall the sense of professional impotence that had emerged so strongly from the nurses' phase 1 data was a less marked feature in the phase 2 accounts.

The boundaries

Although the nurses' phase 2 data reveal some growth in the nurses' personal and professional confidence, there was also evidence, confirmed in the literature, that within health-care practice professional dominance still operates and nurses still experience considerable difficulties in their exercise of professional autonomy (Greenwood 1994).

> It's just knowing the professional boundaries. What we are allowed to say and what we aren't allowed to say. What should be said by us and what should be said by someone else. That's why some of us are still wary about talking to relatives.
>
> Interview no. 7

> The medical staff could be a lot more informative. They go off on a ward round and don't tell the nurse they are about to start it, and make decisions on that ward round that they don't get back to the nurses.
>
> Interview no. 10

> I feel that communication between the nurse, patient and relative is really good now but the medical staff . . . . It always comes down to medical staff. Sometimes we don't go on ward rounds – they go off without us. I find it very hard to approach people who take that view of you.
>
> Interview no. 4

Breaking the mould

In some wards, the nurses had largely succeeded in their efforts to be included with the medical staff in discussions with relatives about the patient's prognosis and diagnosis or, at the very least, to be kept fully informed of the relatives' current understanding and acceptance of their loved one's condition. The following exemplar reveals, however, that success in this area was variable.

> Since this study has been up and running, and we've come back with our standard, we have been able to accost doctors who are about to speak to relatives. It doesn't always work but doctors are beginning to understand that nurses need communication.
>
> Interview no. 3

In two wards where medical staff had cooperated fully with the nurses in their efforts to improve communication, significant benefits were reported.

What we can offer them [relatives] now is continuity of information which we weren't really able to offer before. I have had personal assurances from Doctor S and I have spoken to the other consultants about having a nurse present when diagnosis and prognosis are being given. So there is a continuity of information. And they [doctors] are all very willing.

Interview no. 12

Over the last few months we have made a conscientious effort to be there when the doctors are speaking to the relatives because so often they [relatives] are only taking in about a quarter of what the doctors are saying. If we take in the rest then we can then reiterate for them. I think that is really important.

Interview no. 10

The medical staff are now realizing that this study has been going on and that it's important for us to be there when relatives are spoken to. That has probably been the most significant part of it. That really didn't happen before.

Interview no. 10

Collaborative approach

The above data indicate that, when there is greater collaboration between medical and nursing staff, communication between nurses and relatives can be significantly enhanced. The data also confirm that, when they can feel confident in their own knowledge of relatives' acceptance and understanding of their loved ones' prognosis, this released the nurses from the anxiety that they might inadvertently 'say the wrong thing' or 'be the first to break the bad news'.

The phase 2 data also indicate that some nurses are now undertaking more detailed assessments of the relatives' needs. In response to socioeconomic issues raised in the phase 1 data, several nurses reported making increased referrals to the hospital social worker. Involving other professionals in the care team in this way reflects a more collaborative and holistic approach to the provision of care. The following exemplar illustrates this change.

Another thing we're better at now is involving the social work department. I think at the first interview I said I had never even thought of involving a social worker. A lot more people are hearing about it and they think they'll get in touch as well. I feel we're using them more than we did before.

Interview no. 5

Having considered how interprofessional issues might influence the support that nurses can offer to relatives of dying patients' the focus now shifts to the nurses' own feelings and experiences, particularly with regard to their participation in the current study.

The participants' perspective

When the nurses agreed to become participants in the current study, this represented a considerable undertaking on their part. Their involvement spanned a period of around 18 months during which they had to acquire a range of skills, such as those involved in helping with sample recruitment processes, developing and implementing quality assurance standards, facilitating change within their own teams, and monitoring and evaluating the care that they provide. The impact that the study has had is reported from a range of perspectives.

Effects on facilitators

The phase 2 data reveal the nurses to be confident in their claims for personal and professional growth and improved confidence which they attributed to their involvement in the study. It was possible to subject the nurses' claims of positive change to scrutiny by using the electronic navigation pathways provided by the analysis software and/or by consulting hard copies of the text from different data sets. In this way corroboration could be sought from data from the phase 2 relatives who had received care in the same wards. It was similarly possible to subject a nurse's claims for changes in her perceptions or practice to comparison by consulting phase 1 and phase 2 data from the same nurse. This form of comparative analysis could be achieved using the navigation facility in the software and/or by consulting hard copies of the text from different data sets.

The nurses' claims are well supported in both sets of data and also in their reported changes in career aspirations. At the end of the study, around half of the nurses were currently either seeking entry to or had just started courses of study in palliative care or cancer nursing. Nevertheless, the following exemplars confirm that participation in the study represented a significant challenge to the nurses.

It was the challenge of it all [that felt good]. To begin with, after we decided to do it, and I realized I'd all this to change, I thought 'Am I *ever* going to do it?' I mean it did take time . . . . But now I know everyone is involved and it's good to think 'this wouldn't have happened if we hadn't done this'. Now when you see wee things being done that weren't done before you feel – that was *us* that got this up and running.

Interview no. 5

Initially we wondered if we were getting anywhere. But I have enjoyed doing it, The fear at the beginning – and wondering if you're doing it right – is it working? When I look back on it as a whole I have really benefited.

Interview no. 6

Almost without exception the nurses reported personal and professional growth as a result of their participation in the study. The following quotes are typical of many of the views expressed in this regard.

It's been brilliant. It has opened up a whole new area for me. I mean bereavement is hardly mentioned in training. It's only when you look into it you see that each family is different and that you need to treat them as individuals. I have enjoyed the study. It has been very very useful.

Interview no. 9

I feel privileged to have been part of the study just because as far as I am aware there hasn't been one done like this in Scotland. Obviously that's a privilege and I feel really good about that.

Interview no. 10

When we saw the document [workshop manual] that you had put together and we could hand it to the other girls in the ward to read – just to know that we had been a part of that was really good. And then getting some feedback from the other nurses in the ward . . . that they too felt as you did.

Interview no. 1

Reports of increased confidence and enhanced comfort when dealing with dying patients and their families represented a prominent feature in the nurses' phase 2 data. The reduction in anxiety and the growth in confidence revealed in the quotes below are representative of the comments offered by many nurses in the study.

I feel satisfied. I feel that I am more confident now dealing with it and talking to people. Most of their questions I do feel comfortable with now. Death doesn't seem to be the taboo subject it was. I can talk about death now and it doesn't upset me the way it used to.

Interview no. 14

I have thoroughly enjoyed it. At the beginning I knew very little about research and standard setting. I didn't know if I'd be interested in that but I thought I would see how I got on. I have thoroughly enjoyed it and would love to do something like this in the future. And I feel a lot more positive about patients' relatives now than when you first interviewed me.

Interview no. 12

Impact of the data

In the words of one of the staff nurses the relatives' data 'really packed a punch'. Hearing and reading the relatives' phase 1 accounts was the main reported reason for the nurses' increased awareness of the relatives' needs. The accounts confirmed that the phase 1 research data had acted as a powerful motivator to change. The quote below echoes many other such reports.

I feel as though I've learned a lot about care of relatives. And I thoroughly enjoyed reading through the research data. I just feel as though I've learnt a lot more than I've put in. Although in saying that it was tough at the time and I've enjoyed being involved in it.

Interview no. 6

Impact of the workshop

The workshop proved to be pivotal to the study. It gave substance to what had been somewhat abstract and it provided the nurses with a focus from which the team spirit and sense of solidarity, which was to prove so valuable, could develop. It has already been reported in Chapter 6 that the workshop was very positively evaluated by the nurses. By meeting the other study participants and hearing common anxieties expressed, peer support was provided. The following exemplar confirms the support that accrued from the workshop.

I loved that two-day workshop. It was so nice to meet other people who for years have had exactly the same frustrations as myself. I used to feel so isolated. You realize now there are all those people out there feeling the same and we are all aiming towards the same thing. That was wonderful.

Interview no. 13

Applying insights gained from the data fed back at the workshop into clinical practice required considerable energy from the nurses and also relied heavily on their skills as facilitators and change agents within their own wards. The extent to which the nurses believe that care was influenced by the intervention is considered below. It has already been stated that nurses' claims for positive changes in practice could be verified by accounts from relatives in the same ward.

Impact on care

The phase 2 data suggest that, by developing and implementing the standards and by monitoring and evaluating care, the nurses have taken some control over their practice. The potential that a standard-setting initiative can have for the empowerment of staff nurses has already been reported in the literature (Methot et al. 1992). Adopting such 'problem-focused' approaches proved effective in this difficult situation.

The following exemplars highlight the potential for reciprocal benefits when the nurses applied these insights to their practice.

> I think we make the relatives feel a lot more comfortable now – by being able to offer them a bed to sleep in overnight – which I think has made a really big difference. In fact, even just by saying, 'Please stay. You are very welcome to stay'.
>
> Interview no. 15

> I'm more aware now of what the relatives' needs are. What their anxieties are. I am much more in-tune with them now. You realize that you should make that extra effort to be there for them when they want to speak to you . . . . Because sometimes just two minutes of your time is worth so much to them.
>
> Interview no. 10

The transactional nature of the stress experienced during a terminal illness, and the fact that relatives usually represent the dying patient's primary source of support, was acknowledged by several nurses during their phase 2 interviews. The following exemplar suggests that by augmenting relatives' coping resources the nurse believes that it might also be possible to realize benefits for the dying patient.

> If the relatives feel more comfortable, if we're offering them more support, and making an effort to be more involved with them then I'm sure that must reflect

on to the patient. If you're trying to reduce some of the relatives' anxieties, by having the relatives' room and involving other people . . . . If the relatives feel better it must reflect on the patients.

Interview no. 5

The nurses' own coping resources and the level of support that they received from their ward teams is reported below.

Support and solidarity

As the study progressed, and especially during the intervention period, a 'team spirit' developed to varying degrees in most of the study wards. The data confirm that, when the staff nurse facilitators' efforts met with a shared commitment to change from within the ward team, they gained support from this. In such a climate feelings of isolation were less likely to be reported. The following exemplars represent some of the positive experiences that nurses reported in this area.

I think the other nurses have been very good. Very willing to try things if we sit and explain – and they've given suggestions as well. When we set the standard we spoke to everyone about it as far as we possibly could. They all helped to shape the standard.

Interview no. 3

The sisters have been supportive. At first it was quite difficult to get people to give out letters unless I asked them to, but then the sisters seemed to take it on when we weren't there. People are looking out for suitable relatives. Everyone is participating now.

Interview no. 4

Some members of staff have actually been quite good. It helps if you do get back-up from colleagues. And the medical staff have been involved, which I was surprised at. That's really quite an achievement.

Interview no. 9

These data suggest that change was more likely to be successfully implemented when the staff nurse facilitators worked in collaborative and supportive climates and when they had access to leadership and peer support. The representative quote offered below encapsulates many of the points raised by the nurses in this regard.

> One of the big things all the way through this study was having a leader who was enthusiastic about everything to make us think that maybe there is something here. That, for one, has made me think I am learning and benefiting. And I really appreciated the workshop as well – just knowing there were others there. And having two nurses involved in the ward was a very good idea too.
>
> Interview no. 6

The data suggest that the researcher's professional identity and the comfortable relationships that developed within the study team supported the staff nurses and acted as a buffer when difficulties arose. Some of these difficulties that the nurses encountered as they implemented their standards in the wards are reported below.

Frustrations along the way

The slow pace of change, obstacles and constraints to change, and disappointments about what had not been achieved were all described in the nurses' phase 2 accounts. The most frequently voiced frustrations related to the failure, in some wards, to have secured improvements in facilities for relatives. A few nurses also expressed frustration as a result of perceived lack of support from nursing management. More than half of the nurses also expressed unresolved difficulties in interprofessional communication. Nurses in two of the wards expressed frustration because support from their ward nursing colleagues had been patchy or absent. The nature of these frustrations and the feelings that they engender are revealed in the following exemplars.

> The room. We keep going back to that but it is *really* frustrating. Also I think I've mentioned how it's really frustrating having a consultant who tells the nurses one thing and relatives another. That's very, very frustrating.
>
> Interview no. 10

> Some people are just not interested and they don't back you up. There are maybe relatives that you have missed because somebody didn't want to hand out a letter or didn't even bother because you weren't there.
>
> Interview no. 4

The experiences and feelings that the nurses reported about their involvement in the study often reflected a complex mixture of successes and frustrations similar to those revealed below.

A lot of people were interested in it [the study]. Even the medical staff. It was nice to have it acknowledged that we had written the standard and they had obviously read it which was nice – because they are now aware of the fact that you are doing something. I really had hoped for the relatives' room, which would have been really good. But that never happened.

Interview no. 2

The analysis of the staff nurses' phase 2 interviews is concluded using a quote from one of the participating nurses.

If we hadn't done this study God knows when this issue would have been dealt with. Well it has been dealt with now. We have it in black and white. This is our standard and it has to be achieved. Obviously the standard of care will improve.

Interview no. 12

Chapter 9
Evaluation

Difficulties in evaluating planned change initiatives within an action setting are well documented (Titchen and Binnie 1993; Greenwood 1994; Lutjens and Tiffany 1994). In particular Greenwood (1994) recommends using a range of approaches and tools, and she advocates seeking the insiders' perspective when evaluating an applied research initiative. Accordingly, this chapter seeks to consider some of the findings of the study from a range of different perspectives. First, the standard evaluation data collected by the nurses during the standard implementation period are reported and discussed, and their congruence with the findings from the phase 2 nurses' and relatives' interview data assessed. The researcher's judgements about the magnitude of change that occurred in relation to different aspects of attempted change in the study wards are then offered. Finally, some major issues and insights to emerge from the interpretation of the nurses' and the relatives' interview data are examined using the device of brief paradigm cases which are presented with interpretative comment.

Evaluation of the standards

Quality assurance standards represented the mechanism for implementing the changes during the intervention period in the current study. This decision was taken because it was judged likely that this approach would be familiar to the staff nurses and also because a standard-setting initiative can incorporate an evaluation strategy.

An unforeseen difficulty was that the scope of attempted change, and the need for extensive consultation, meant that getting the standards to the stage of implementation took around 7 months and involved much effort from all concerned. Some of the results of those efforts have already been reported in the relatives' and nurses' interview data presented in Chapters 7 and 8. Attention is now directed towards the evaluation data collected by the *staff nurses* on an ongoing basis during the period when the standards were being implemented in their wards. Findings reported here therefore represent the *nurses' judgements* about achievement of the standard criteria.

It has already been established that the development and implementation of the standards represented a 'bottom-up' ward-based initiative (Harvey 1994). Although this approach brought all the benefits of ownership, the completed standards lacked uniformity, making evaluation problematic. Also, although it was judged important that the content and scope of the standards were wholly determined by the nurses, the researcher did provide assistance with the layout and typing of the standards and with the development of a 'Standard Evaluation Tool' for each individual standard.

The evaluation tools were designed to monitor achievement of a combination of structure, process and outcome criteria. It was intended that the emerging data from this initiative would facilitate ongoing, formative evaluation of care at ward level, so that achievement or non-achievement of criteria could be monitored, and acted upon, by the ward nurses. Collation of these standard evaluation data would also contribute to the final summative evaluation of the impact of the change. A 'Clinical Standard Record of Use' form was also provided to enable the nurses to record how often the standard was applied with families in the ward and to allow problems encountered by the staff during implementation of the standard to be monitored and recorded.

Collated evaluations of clinical standards

A total of 79 completed evaluations forms were submitted at the end of the phase 2 recruitment period. Nurses in the study wards were asked to complete an evaluation form (see Appendix 1) each time the standard was applied with the family of a dying patient. Compliance with this request was variable. In some wards the standard was evaluated with the family of every dying patient, whereas in others evaluations were submitted only for those families who were recruited into the study. In one ward the standard was never implemented and consequently no evaluations were submitted.

Following the workshop at which the phase 1 data were presented and draft standards were drawn up, the staff nurses worked with their nursing teams to complete the development of their own standard. Although there were broad similarities in the areas that staff in the different wards chose to address, differences in wording and in the numerical codes used in the standard criteria and accompanying evaluation tools precluded direct ward-by-ward comparison. Furthermore, although some wards provided quite detailed information in their evaluation documents, others supplied minimal data indicating achievement/non-achievement merely by a 'yes/no' or a tick.

Steps taken to collate the evaluation data are:

- Evaluations were first collated for each ward.
- Individual evaluations from each ward were then scrutinized.
- Areas of achievement and non-achievement of the standard criteria were identified and recorded.
- Percentage level of non-achievement was calculated for (1) each single family, (2) overall for each ward and (3) across all of the study wards.
- Written comments offered by the nurses were then collated.

Collated standard evaluation data are summarized in Table 19.1.

Evidence from the collated data suggests that efforts to improve family care have met with a fair measure of success. Improvements in facilities were achieved in a number of wards. However, in two wards, despite efforts made by the participating nurses to secure improvements in facilities for relatives, none was achieved. Comments in the evaluation forms from these wards refer to lack of privacy during communication and one situation is described when the privacy and support needs of a distressed relative were unmet as a result of lack of suitable accommodation.

Improvements were frequently recorded in the area of communication. Efforts to improve relatives' access to nursing staff appeared to be largely successful. Improved communications within the nursing team were also achieved. It is now reported to be 'usual practice' during the report to discuss the relatives' support needs and their awareness of and response to the patient's prognosis. Evaluation data also suggest that interprofessional communication has improved in some wards but remains problematic in others.

Table 9.1: Collated evaluations of clinical standards

Hospital/ward	Number of completed evaluations submitted	Number criteria assessed per evaluation	Overall criteria achieved per ward (%)	Area of non-achievement identified	Reason given for non-achievement	Comments offered
A1	7	8	98	Privacy during communication	No private area available	Distressed relative in corridor when duty room was occupied
A2	10	11	95	Interprofessional communication	Occasions when no record made of doctor–relative information exchange	Nurse/doctor communication still less than adequate at times
				Support around time of death	Patient's rapid deterioration prevented full family support	
A3	20	7	90	Privacy during communication	No private area available	Duty room was only available place and was open to interruption
B1	4	11	100			
B2	0				The standard was never implemented in this ward	
B3	34	12	76	Interprofessional communication	Including nurses in information. Exchange now happens more often but is not yet a *fully* established practice	*Very* detailed evaluations submitted. Nurse/medical communication now very much improved
B4	4	10	95	Support around time of death	Rapid deterioration in patients' condition at times precluded full implementation	Evaluation difficult – as staff and patients re-located twice during standard implementation period

Number of evaluations conducted = 79; Average % criteria achievement overall = 92%

The nurses used the comments section of the evaluation tool to highlight their own difficulties when trying to recruit relatives for the phase 2 sample. Reasons (with frequency) for non-recruitment of relatives are summarized below:

- Patient still on active treatment (1)
- Rapid deterioration in patient's condition (12)
- Patient transferred to hospice/home (8)
- Relatives too distressed/unable to accept prognosis (9)
- Difficult family dynamics (3)
- Relative not in attendance (2).

It must be acknowledged that the evaluation procedures adopted by the nurses were outwith the researcher's direct control. Consequently, no firm claims can be made for the validity of these data. However, the data do offer revealing insight into the nurses' difficulties and achievements as they strove to secure improved care for families of dying patients in their wards. The evaluation process also underscored the benefits of adopting a reflective analytical approach to nursing practice.

Area and magnitude of change

Judgements made about the areas of change that were attempted, and the magnitude of change that had occurred in relation to these different aspects of practice, drew on data from a range of sources. This included phase 2 interview data from both nurses and relatives, staff nurses' post-workshop evaluation, completed clinical standard evaluation documents, and the researcher's observations and copious field notes.

Using evaluation data from a range of sources allowed for some measure of cross-validation of findings and permitted the evidence of change to be viewed from a number of different perspectives. It has already been reported in Chapters 4 and 8 that the corroboration of findings was greatly facilitated by the electronic navigation features of the analysis software (Padilla 1993), e.g. if reports were made in the nurses' phase 2 interview data that it is now 'usual practice' for the nurses to initiate and maintain regular contact with the family, it was possible to seek further evidence that this practice was indeed being applied by consulting the relatives' phase 2 interview data. Similarly, if a nurse claimed that she now felt more comfortable when communicating with the dying patient's family, by returning to her phase 1 account, it was possible to establish what her reported experiences and feelings in this area had been in the pre-intervention period.

Moreover, if data from the standard evaluation documents indicated achievement of the criteria in relation to nurse–relative communication, by checking this finding against both sets of interview data it was possible to confirm whether the recorded change was reflected in the relatives' and the nurses' experiences reported during the interview.

The comments that follow relate to the magnitude of change achieved by different ward teams, in relation to different *aspects* of the change initiative (such as the provision of a private area for relatives).

Recording of these judgements used the following nomenclature:

(Ma) = major change occurred
(Mo) = moderate change occurred and
(Mi) = minimal or no change occurred.

It must be stressed that the judgements offered relate to recorded, reported or observed *evidence of actual change* and do not represent a judgement about the effort invested in attempting change, e.g. in relation to acquiring or upgrading a room for the relatives, (Ma) suggests that structural or other substantial modification took place, (Mo) indicates that an existing room was upgraded whereas (Mi) suggests that no change or very little change in provision had occurred – often despite energetic efforts on the part of the nurses to improve this aspect of care.

In relation to the category 'medical/nursing communication', (Ma) indicates that substantial changes in practice had been established. An example of a major change in practice in this area might be that a nurse now routinely accompanies medical staff during interviews with the family. (Mo) suggests that some change was achieved in this area but that this was rather less than had been hoped for by the nurses. An example of moderate change might be

that, although doctors sometimes 'forget' to include nurses in interviews with families, they do now regularly inform nursing staff of the
relatives' current awareness and of the outcome of meetings that
they have had with the family. Finally, (Mi) indicates that there was
no real evidence of change in this area – again often despite the
nurses' efforts to improve this aspect of care.

Although the subjective nature of these change magnitude data is
fully acknowledged, they do offer some insight into overall patterns
of change both within and between wards, and they allow the
researcher's observations and judgements to be reported. Evidence
suggests that the greatest magnitude of change overall occurred in
wards that had successfully implemented measures to provide, or
upgrade, a room where the relatives could rest and where they could
receive information, counselling and support in privacy and
comfort. It has already been reported in Chapter 8 that, when nurses
achieved change in this crucial area, other positive changes tended
to follow.

One seemingly modest change in terms of resources was the
provision of a camp bed, yet, for relatives who were involved in staying overnight at the bedside, this drew frequent positive comment.
However, undoubtedly the most notable change was in the
frequency of reports in both the nurses' and the relatives' phase 2
data about the reciprocal benefits that resulted from the more
relaxed climate that characterized relationships between relatives
and nurses in most of the study wards.

Review of the major themes

The focus now shifts to adopt a slightly different perspective, in order
to review some major themes that emerged from both the relatives'
and the nurses' interview data. First, to explore the phase 2 relatives'
experiences, three brief paradigm cases are presented and comment
on the issues that emerge from these offered. One paradigm case
selected from the nurses' accounts is then presented and the issues
that emerge from this inform discussion of the impact of the study on
the participating nurse from both a personal and a professional
perspective.

Relatives' paradigm no. 1

'Vigil supported'

Background

Jan is a 40-year-old school teacher and mother of two children aged 7 and 9. Over the past week, she has been staying in the ward most of the day and also overnight with her dying mother. When her mother was admitted to hospital last week with acute breathing diffi-culties, her death looked imminent. At the time of interview, although her mother's condition remained very poor, it had stabilized somewhat. The text below represents the dialogue that took place when Jan was asked about her experiences while in the ward and during her overnight stays.

Researcher: How often are you visiting at the moment, Jan?

Jan: I'm here more or less all of the time. Ken [patient's partner] and I are taking it turn about to stay overnight. I try to be here as much as possible. I've been off work all of last week, but I intend going back tomorrow morning. I'll stay overnight and then go to work straight from here tomorrow. I'm a school teacher and I've got classes and they [pupils] are only a few weeks away from exams. Even if it's only for a couple of hours I'll go in to school to take some classes. The head teacher and all the rest of the staff are very helpful and under-standing. I can come and go as I please. But I do feel that I want to go in. And I know that I can get back here quickly if I need to. Next week I intend to come backwards and forwards [to the hospital] and go in to work in between.

Researcher: When you are here in the ward how welcome and comfortable do you feel?

Jan: I feel very very welcome and very comfortable. The surroundings are pleasant and the nurses are all very cheerful and understanding. They can't do enough for you.

Researcher: What are they doing that you find helpful?

Jan: Well, they [the nurses] are talking to me. They are asking me how my mum is and asking how *I* am. I would say over the past few days that they are concen-trating more on me . . . well maybe not *more* on me, but just as much on me and my well-being as caring for my mother.

Researcher: How does that feel?

Jan: It makes me feel really good. Really secure. They're excellent . . . giving you cups of tea and coffee.

Researcher: When you stayed overnight in the ward how comfortable were you?

Jan: Very comfortable. As long as my mother is settled and sleeps through the whole night, I can sleep through the whole night as well.

Researcher: How are you managing that. I mean where are you sleeping?

Jan: I am sleeping on a Z-Bed in beside her. Right in beside her, next to her bed. There has only been one night that I didn't sleep at all. But that was because my mother was very disturbed that night. The other nights she has been settled all night and I have slept all night. In fact on Saturday morning we didn't get up until 8.45 [laughter]. I haven't slept to that time at home. My husband and I have obviously talked about my mother's condition and we are both pretty aware that the majority of people die through the night . . . and I would just hate her to be alone. So it's good. I feel better knowing that I can be here through the night.

Interview no. 2/13

Comment

In some respects Jan offers a 'typical' example of the female relatives who featured prominently in both relatives' samples in this study, in that she is faced with the competing demands of children, work and a dying relative. The second paragraph in the exemplar reveals Jan's inner conflict as she tries to respond to the rival claims that are being made on her.

Jan was able to call on a number of coping resources to help her deal with these difficulties. As her husband worked from home, this relieved her of some of the worry associated with the home and children. She also enjoyed a mutually supportive relationship with her husband that proved crucial to her coping efforts. Jan is also a professional woman who enjoys a fair degree of autonomy and can rely on supportive relationships at work and has the security of knowing that she need not fear for her job. Nevertheless, her own sense of commitment creates a degree of tension which she clearly planned to resolve by dividing her time up between work and hospital. Jan's effective network of social support confirms findings in the literature that middle-class, well-educated people generally have better access to coping resources and are thus able to employ more efficacious (problem-focused) coping strategies (Pearlin and Schooler 1978).

Issues to emerge from Jan's experiences in the ward relate mainly to the emotional climate in the ward and to factors within the ward environment. Jan clearly feels comfortable and accepted in the ward because she describes how the nurses talk to her and show concern for her well-being. A connection has clearly been established between Jan and the nurses, and the effect of this is expressed as 'I feel secure' thus confirming the nurturing potential of such relationships. Moreover, in that ward climate Jan is clearly free from any concern about feeling like 'a nuisance' or of being 'in the way'.

Facilities provided for Jan's comfort during her long vigil also helped her to cope with the situation. She describes feeling well rested and comfortable, which contrasts with the overwhelming exhaustion reported by most relatives in phase 1 and by around a third of the phase 2 relatives. The support she derived from being able to remain physically close to her mother is also evident as Jan repeats the phrase 'I'm right in beside her'. Reports that relatives derive support from being comfortably accommodated close to their dying loved one have emerged consistently in the data in the current study and have also been reported in the literature (Hull 1989a).

Although facilities for physical comfort such as a bed, a room to rest in and regular refreshments in themselves represent 'palliative' measures, the support that they provided strengthened this relative's coping efforts at a time when coping resources might have been severely taxed. Indeed, in Jan's case, being able to sleep in comfort alongside her mother relieved her stress and also ensured that she was sufficiently rested to make plans to accommodate her professional commitments. Thus, for Jan these interventions facilitated the use of problem-focused coping strategies.

Finally, by facilitating contact between the dying patient and family in these final days, there might be potential to reduce future regret in grieving relatives.

Jan sums up *her* feelings thus 'I would just hate her to be alone. I feel better knowing that I can be here'.

Relatives' paradigm no. 2

Facing it together

Background

Mrs Brown (prefers Ethel) is 75 years old and somewhat frail. She has twice had surgery in the past year. One operation was for a prolapsed uterus, the other to correct a foot problem. Ethel's 76-year-old husband Bill is dying. Although still mentally alert, Bill's physical condition is deteriorating and he is becoming aware of this. The exemplar below was selected because it offers revealing insight into some of the complex issues inherent in the transition from an awareness context, where staff and relatives collude to conceal the diagnosis from the patient, to a situation of open disclosure.

Ethel: My neighbour had come up to see my husband and when she asked him how he was feeling he said, 'I'd feel better if they'd tell me the truth. They're all just humming and hawing around it and I know there's something more going on. But I'm just getting wee snatches here and there.' He was putting two and two together and getting eight. You know? So I said to him, 'Well – would you really like to know, Bill?' and he said 'Aye. I would. I really would like to know the truth.'

So I took my neighbour round to the lift and who was coming off the lift but Bill's doctor. The doctor put his arm around my shoulder and he said 'How are you coping Mrs Brown?' [control slipping – becoming tearful]. I said: 'Not too bad doctor but the only thing is Bill wants to know the truth.' The doctor said 'Well if you feel you can tell him then you do that and I'll come right round.' So I did it and we both had a wee bubble and then the doctor came in and he spoke to us both. [weeping freely throughout]

Researcher: That was a very brave but a very difficult thing to do . . . .

Ethel: The doctor was so nice and gentle. He's a real gentleman . . . .

Researcher: How was Bill after you had told him and you both had your cry together?

Ethel: Well, then the doctor came in and I said to him, 'I've told him, doctor . . .' Now he [Bill] just sits and stares into space and when I say to him 'What are you thinking about Bill?', he says 'Everything and nothing.' Och aye. But I think he'll cope all right [sighs].'

Interview no. 2/17

Comment

The above exemplar highlights the very common situation, also reported in the literature, where relatives are told the prognosis but the patient is not (Seale 1991; Steptoe et al. 1991). Issues involved in collusion of this nature are poignantly revealed in Ethel's account.

As Bill's suspicions about his deteriorating health grew he voiced these through the safe medium of a third party (a neighbour), thereby giving Ethel the option to either pick-up on the cue or to let it pass. Ethel, who clearly knew Bill better than anyone else could, decided to act on his signal and to take on the difficult task of disclosing the grave prognosis. In the above account, Ethel's strength (despite her apparent frailty) and the sensitivity of the doctor stand out sharply.

The doctor responded sensitively to Ethel's obvious distress when they met at the lift. He respected the couple's need for privacy during the disclosure but also appreciated their subsequent need for the support from a caring third party.

The enormity of the disclosure clearly had a major impact on Bill. This confirms that, even when a patient is seemingly suspicious about their prognosis, denial can still operate as a potent defence and hopes of recovery might still be harboured. As Bill absorbed the impact, he became quiet and withdrawn, and Ethel clearly felt that she couldn't reach him – 'he just sits and stares into space now'. During this part of the interview Ethel's demeanour was bleak and she was weeping quietly. Nevertheless, she expressed confidence that Bill would recover from the blow, 'Aye . . . but I think he'll cope with it all right'.

This couple's close, loving relationship had spanned some 52 years and respect for Bill's right to the truth and her own discomfort with the continuing deception led Ethel to act on the cue that her husband had offered.

Hinton (1981), in a study of collusion in spouses, noted that couples caught up in such deception were unable to comfort one another and as a result each partner was left to bear their pain alone. Ethel and Bill faced it together.

Relatives' paradigm no. 3

Vigil disturbed

Background

At the time of this interview David, aged 72, was sitting with his wife Margaret, who died the day after the interview. In his otherwise very positive account, David reported stress that both he and Margaret had experienced as a result of being in the midst of the noise and bustle of a busy surgical ward. In an exemplar presented in Chapter 7, David described the stress experienced while sitting at his dying wife's bedside in a four-bedded room with televisions on and other patients' children running around. The data below represent David's response when asked at the end of the interview, 'Is there anything that you would like to add before we finish?'

> *David*: Well . . . I know it's awful stupid but there was a nurse going down the corridor the other night and the trolley was squeaking like billy-ho and the door was open because my wife was feeling claustrophobic . . . .
>
> *Researcher*: Are you saying that loud noises . . .?
>
> *David*: *Yes* . . . And another thing I would say is that the nurses' station is directly opposite her room door and they keep all the case notes in a trolley right beside her door. And the clerkess has peerie [stiletto] heels on . . . I mean *you* might not hear it but for me . . . for Margaret . . . . You can *see* her getting distressed with the noise. Also, the nurses are nice young lassies but they *do* talk and have the odd wee giggle. What I would like to see is an island nurses' station with just enough glass up so that the noise is kept inside – and the files are all kept in there too. [all said very gently]
>
> *Researcher*: I take your point David. You are in a hub of activity just when you want to be at your most peaceful with Margaret.
>
> Interview no. 2/5

Comment

These data emphasize the needs that dying patients and their relatives have to be in an environment that is free from intrusive distractions and yet that offers regular support and attention from staff. By convention, dying patients in hospital tend to be located next to the nurses' station to allow maximum observation and contact. Although the logic in this is persuasive, disadvantages were revealed in this account. Sharp insight into the relatives' perspective about the nature of the vigil emerged from these data. An impression emerged of David 'standing guard' over Margaret and seeking to secure an appropriate and respectful 'dying space' for his wife.

These three brief paradigm cases have focused on major themes to emerge from the relatives' phase 2 analysis. In the first, the relative (Jan) was experiencing the benefits of relatively modest environmental changes that had been made by the nurses and of the excellent efforts made by the staff to create an emotional climate where relatives could feel welcome and supported in the ward. The wider benefits to relatives of these coping supports were also revealed in Jan's account.

The second paradigm adopted the relative's (Ethel's) perspective on some of the complex issues that surround collusion and disclosure of prognosis. This paradigm was included for the revealing insights it offers. In Ethel's account the reciprocal character of hope, and indeed loss of hope, was revealed. On this occasion the professional carer who encountered Ethel in her distress and who offered support was a doctor. It might just as easily have been a nurse and the issues raised are salient.

The third brief paradigm highlighted the specific needs that some patients and relatives have as death draws near. Some of the unresolved difficulties associated with meeting those needs within the context of an acute hospital setting were vividly revealed. All three paradigms adopted a slightly different perspective, but each illustrates the need for the dying patient's family to receive supportive physical and emotional care within an appropriate and welcoming ward environment.

Attention is now directed towards some of the effects of the study on the participating nurses.

Only one nurses' paradigm case is presented for comment. This reflects the salience and comprehensiveness of the exemplar as a focus for discussion of some key issues to emerge from the nurses' data. Although these data describe a unique situation, they also exemplify the commonly reported shifts that occurred in the thinking and in the behaviour of the participating nurses.

Staff nurse paradigm

Advocacy in action

Background

Sue has been in her current post as a senior staff nurse in an acute surgical ward for 5 years. Below she describes her recent experiences when dealing with a terminally ill young man and his wife.

> *Sue*: We had a chap the other week. He was only thirty. That's the youngest I've ever come across. He was only in the ward about a fortnight and I felt the standard really helped us then – because everyone was pushing for this guy to get a bed in the hospice where he should be, because this is such a busy ward.
>
> It was his wife that I really got to know well. They had a wee girl who was only one year old. She [the wife] said to me 'What am I going to do when he dies?' and I said 'I don't know what to say to you . . . but I'll just sit here and be

with you'. She was trying to be so brave and then one night from being in very full control of herself she just cracked completely . . . . That's still hard . . . .

Researcher: How did you deal with it?

Sue: I think I said that it was obviously going to be very hard and I think I spoke more about the wee girl. The family had coped with death so many times that I think she felt that she knew what she was doing because she had been through it all before . . . . And then she realized that before she had always had Tom there with her . . . to go through it with her. It was so sudden. Just six weeks from diagnosis.

Researcher: That must have been really hard.

Sue: Yes. I think it's the worst I've ever been involved with. I think it's the younger age factor [that makes it so stressful?]. I felt the medical staff were holding back . . . so I phoned the man's GP and suggested that he phone the hospice and explain the situation. Before this [study participation] I would never have done that. But they were getting nowhere and his wife was getting so upset at the end. She just couldn't cope with the way he was . . . I arranged for her to go up and see the hospice. Before, I don't think I would have taken all that on and gone ahead and done it.

Researcher: How did it feel for you to do that?

Sue: I felt she really appreciated it. She used to phone and ask for me by name. Before, I would never have got on the phone to the hospice.

Researcher: What gave you the courage?

Sue: He was so young. I felt I had to do something. You couldn't have that man in a busy surgical ward like this. He'd been there for 2 weeks and you could see over the days that there was no way anything was going to cure him.

I was quite proud of myself really. After I phoned the hospice someone came out to see him and we got him in. I kept saying to myself 'I'm overstepping the mark here'. But for him something *had* to be done.

Interview no. 5

Comment

This offers a vivid example of the empowerment that can come from a caring relationship, and it confirms that engagement and involvement can motivate nurses to intercede for patients and families. The growth in confidence and the level of professional autonomy that prompted Sue to act on this young family's behalf are evident in these data.

Several factors might have been at work within this situation. The dying patient (Tom) and his wife (Kim) were close in age to Sue, and the level of identification that nurses can experience when caring for dying patients of a comparable age has been found to result in increased stress (Field and Kitson 1986). Also Sue and Kim had developed an emotional bond. This was evident when Sue said 'it was his wife that I got to know really well'. The transactional character of the relationship is revealed when Sue states 'she would always ask for me by name.' Evidence in the literature reveals that the reciprocal energy generated by such relationships can act as a motivating and empowering force for nurses (Benner and Wrubel 1989; Oberle and Davies 1993).

Sue's reflections revealed her to be both surprised and pleased by her own professional growth. Her increased feelings of self-efficacy and control and an enhanced self-concept were revealed when she said 'I felt I had to do something' and 'I felt quite proud of myself really.' It has been found that such feelings of personal satisfaction are experienced when nurses provide care that is congruent with their own beliefs and values (Oberle and Davies 1993).

Sue also commented that 'having the standard really helped us' and she repeatedly placed her current feelings and behaviour in a comparative (pre-study) context, thus underlining the benefits she perceived that she had gained from her participation in the design and implementation of the standard. The empowerment and sense of ownership and commitment that this type of involvement generated in Sue have also been reported in the literature on quality assurance (Methot et al. 1992).

Although the data clearly reveal Sue's sensitivity to this family's needs, she also confronts and accepts the limitations of what she can realistically offer. She recognizes that to be present with Kim in her distress without further intervention was a valid and comforting action. This insight is powerfully revealed when Sue says to Kim 'I don't know what to say to you . . . but I'll just sit here and be with you'. Sue intuitively recognized the potent power of 'presence' and what it really means to 'be with' another in a connected and empathic way.

Regrettably, the exemplar offers no evidence of interprofessional collaboration; indeed the nurses' and doctors' perception of the problem seemed to differ markedly. Sue confirmed this when she said 'I felt the medical staff were holding back' (and) 'I had to do something because I felt they were getting nowhere'. The nurse–doctor relationships (or absence of relationship) reflect a

medical-dominated context that is familiar to, and has created difficulties for, many nurses who work in hospitals. These difficulties
were revealed in data from both phases of the current study and have
also been reported in the literature (Gibson 1991; Dwyer et al. 1992;
Maslin-Prothero 1992).

By expediting Tom's hospice admission without further recourse
to her medical colleagues, Sue stepped outside the usual confines of
her perceived sphere of 'authority'. As a result of her actions the
family's wishes for a hospice bed were met. However, as the quote
below clearly reveals, although Sue was spurred on to act as she did
out of her concern for this family, the significant underlying interprofessional issues within this situation remain unresolved.

> I kept saying to myself 'I'm overstepping the mark here'. But for him – some-
> thing *had* to be done.

Difficulties so cogently expressed by Sue are echoed in the literature. Greenwood (1994) refers to the psychosocial costs inherent in
research that involves nurses. The author asserts that nurses do not
enjoy any real autonomy in interdisciplinary hospital practice and
she highlights the difficulties that nurses can experience when seeking to implement 'even small-scale innovation' in an environment
that is dominated by other, more powerful, health-care professionals
(Greenwood 1994).

Conclusion

These four paradigm cases each offer something to illuminate the
experience of being a relative of a dying patient in hospital and of
what it means to provide nursing support for such families. 'Vigil
supported' reveals the benefits that relatives derive from a welcoming and friendly ward environment and from access to facilities for
comfort and rest. 'Facing it together' offers insight into the complexities of collusion and reveals the poignant and reciprocal qualities of
hope. 'Vigil disturbed' reveals the stress that both patient and relative
can experience when the 'dying space' is invaded by intrusive
reminders of normality. Finally 'Advocacy in action' offers the
nurses' perspective on the provision of family-focused care and
reveals the effects that advocacy-driven behaviour can have for the
nurse, the patient and the family.

Collectively these data address the major issues raised by the nurses and the relatives, and they reflect a number of key themes that emerged from the analysis. They also reveal areas where change has occurred and areas that have proved resistant to change.

The most powerful message to emerge was that, although stress associated with the impending loss of a loved one is not amenable to amelioration, the coping efforts of both relatives and nurses can be supported by relaxed and warm interpersonal relationships and by environmental resources that promote comfort and privacy and that facilitate communication.

Chapter 10
Discussion, conclusions and recommendations

The chapter is in several sections. First, the choice of research method and the extent to which the approaches used for data gathering and analysis proved appropriate for meeting the aims of the study are reviewed. The aptness of the theoretical framework for exploring, explicating and reporting the experiences and concerns of the relatives and the nurses is then examined. The approach selected for designing, implementing and evaluating the intervention is reviewed and issues pertaining to the planned change initiative discussed. In this discussion, particular reference is made to those factors noted to have facilitated change and those found to have presented barriers to change. In the final section, some conclusions are drawn, the limitations of the study acknowledged, and recommendations for practice and for further research in this area suggested.

Review of the interview approach

Qualitative methods were selected to gather and analyse the data in this study because it was judged that such an approach would allow the respondents the fullest possible opportunity to express their concerns and views in a way that was contextual and that facilitated reciprocal dialogue and clarification. Although proponents of triangulation persuasively argue that fuller understanding might be gained by combining quantitative and qualitative approaches (Goodwin and Goodwin 1984; Corner 1991a), others advocate a more committed adherence to one or other philosophical perspective (Leininger 1984; Parse 1995). In the current study, however,

210

given the very sensitive nature of this investigation, it was judged that the aims of the study could best be met by adhering to a qualitative framework.

The interview approach

The semi-structured interview approach enabled themes derived from the literature to be pursued in a particularly detailed way. Although the questions were mainly of the open variety, and were structured to explore feelings, the instruments were nevertheless more structured than is usual with this approach. It was judged that this instruments' format would provide a basis for comparison of pre- and post-intervention data which might have proved more diffi-cult with an open interview approach. It should also be emphasized that, although the layout of the instruments might suggest that a somewhat tightly structured interview approach had been adopted, this would not fairly or accurately reflect the way in which the instru-ments were delivered, or the relaxed and facilitative emotional climate that characterized most of the interactions.

Questions were organized into sections representing the main themes to be explored. At the end of each section, and again before concluding the interview, respondents were encouraged to add to, or expand upon, what had previously been said. This invitation was very commonly accepted. With increasing skill and confidence, the instruments became a flexible framework around which the main themes were explored and the probes, in italics, were used mainly for re-focusing or as a reflection or clarification device.

Advantages of the structure of the instruments became apparent when entering the pilot study data into the analysis package (Padilla 1993), and subsequently when isolating and manipulating data during the analysis processes. Conducting the 10 pilot study inter-views had also enabled some fluency in interviewing technique to be developed and established that the instruments, as delivered, facili-tated comfortable dialogue from which copious and rich data emerged. This supported the decision to retain the general structure of the instruments, apart from minor reordering of questions to allow a more natural 'conversational' flow and the inclusion of an addi-tional question to allow socioeconomic factors during terminal illness to be explored with the relatives.

Sampling issues

A study of this nature, where the focus of enquiry is in an emotionally sensitive area, clearly relies on cooperation from those who are willing to share their experiences, views and feelings. The potential for sampling bias that this implies was acknowledged in Chapter 4 and also in Chapter 9, where it was also reported that some nurses had found it difficult to approach relatives whom they perceived to be particularly angry, or whose distress was of such magnitude that an approach would have been judged to be insensitive. It is possible that the nurses' selection strategies might have reduced the opportunities to explore issues of interest, or to assess the extent to which the intervention had assisted those relatives judged to be 'difficult' to approach or to be otherwise unsuitable.

Moreover, although the method of introducing the study was well accepted by relatives, the nurses clearly encountered difficulties in identifying the point at which they should offer relatives a letter from the researcher. From discussions with the nurses during ward visits, a strong impression emerged that, even when a patient's condition clearly seemed to place his or her relatives within the sample inclusion criteria, nurses seemed to experience difficulties in accepting that the patient was indeed quite so close to death.

A complex form of professional denial seemed to be at work, with nurses demonstrating, and indeed expressing, a personal reluctance to 'give up on the patient' too soon. This closely parallels the tenacity of hope illustrated in the relatives' data and it seems to support the notion that acknowledgement of the forthcoming death requires a shift in emotional orientation to the patient which nurses might understandably resist. Buchan (1995) has also identified nurses' difficulties in estimating patients' prognoses during the last days of life.

The implications that such professional denial might have for care and support for dying patients and their families, and the nature of the difficulties that nurses experience in assessing the imminence of death, merit further investigation. Also, in situations where the illness took a steep downward trajectory, relatives tended to be around the ward over a briefer time span, thus making it difficult to recruit them into the sample. These difficulties, coupled with the unpredictable nature of the situation, meant that acquiring the relatives' samples took much longer than expected. Measures taken to address these recruitment difficulties and to analyse them included maintenance of a researcher's 'ward contact log' to allow sampling patterns and difficulties across the eight studies to be monitored, and a 'sample recruitment log' which the nurses completed each week so that the number of deaths that had occurred during the past week, and the number of patients currently receiving 'terminal care' within the ward, could be recorded.

Review of the analysis approach

In the pilot study, and during the very early stages of the phase 1 analysis, a structured analysis approach was adopted. At this point the study was being conducted within the framework of an evaluation research design and the approach to analysis followed a fairly structured approach using the coding and classification framework that had been developed from the pilot study.

However, as analysis progressed, and insights and interpretative skills were gained, the richness and power of the data led to a growing dissonance with this analysis approach. Compelling themes, such as 'hope' and 'reciprocity', which were emerging from the data, fuelled a search for deeper understanding that moved the analyst into an increasingly engaged and absorbed interpretative relationship with the data; this also led to a further search for insight by consulting extant theory and the literature.

The interpretative processes that subsequently drove the enquiry forward were greatly facilitated by the analysis software, which permitted ease of movement between text segments and their source data and allowed linkages and associations with biographical data and between different data sets to be explored. The cyclical and deepening character of the analysis, which involved the identification and interpretation of themes, exemplars and paradigm cases, showed clear parallels with the hermeneutic textual analysis approach (Kvale 1983; Reinharz 1983; Reeder 1987; Leonard 1989). In essence, the impact of these data and the researcher's increasing sensitivity to the text caused the analysis to evolve from a descriptive approach to a cyclical, thematic and reflexive interpretative approach in the hermeneutic tradition.

Qualms about embracing the complex philosophies associated with this analysis approach were somewhat allayed, after reference to the works of a number of nurse scholars who had espoused the hermeneutic method and had usefully placed it within the context of nursing practice (Leininger 1984; Reeder 1988; Sandelowski 1991; Thorne 1991; Walters 1994). Phenomenology's respect for subjective reality, and for the uniqueness of each person's experience, sits comfortably with the humanistic approach to nursing that embraces individuality and holism. Indeed when nurses seek to empathize with individual patients and clients, they could be said to be bringing a 'phenomenological attitude' to their practice (Thorne 1991; Walters 1994).

Moreover, some of the philosophical tensions that cause concern to committed phenomenologists, e.g. accepting individual uniqueness while acknowledging shared realities, are not so relevant within the highly contextualized world of nursing. Nurse phenomenologists, rather than searching deeply for unique 'being', are more likely to apply the hermeneutic approach to illuminate common elements within subjective experiences. In this respect hermeneutic research and nursing practice show close parallels. The hermeneutic circle is manifest within the commonplace and everyday 'worlds' of nursing practice where, in their caring practice, nurses strive to comprehend the whole by relating the parts to the whole as they attend to the myriad factors that influence the comfort and the well-being of those for whom they care. The current study, although not claiming to follow all of the tenets of the hermeneutic method, was approached with a 'phenomenological attitude' which acknowledged the primacy of the subjective experience, the obligation to respect the unique qualities of each respondent and the accounts that they offered, and the duty to use insights gained from the study to support good professional practice.

The data-gathering methods used in the current study, and in particular the interpretative approach that was ultimately adopted, offered an appropriate strategy for meeting the aims of the study and for doing so from a holistic and humanistic perspective.

The utility of such an approach for influencing nursing practice is encapsulated in the following quote.

> It seems crucial to illuminate through hermeneutics the persistent and enduring
> values of our discipline that empower, emancipate and impassion human
> caring and that awakens sensitivity to our shared human condition. Respect
> and the skilful use of language is one of our most human of expressions in
> pursuit of these goals.
>
> (Reeder 1988, p. 229)

Review of the theoretical framework

The cognitive, phenomenological, transactional model of stress and coping as explicated by Wrubel et al. (1981) was adopted as the theoretical framework for the current study.

In the wholly cognitive view of stress, the mind is seen as being rather like a rational calculator that operates distinct from and distant to the external world. From this somewhat unitary perspective, successful coping represents mastery, control and rationality. However, in situations such as terminal illness, mastery, control and rationality are not usually viable options (Benner and Wrubel 1989). In contrast, the cognitive, phenomenological, transactional perspective recognizes that, although coping might include cognitive processes, it cannot be seen purely in terms of an unlimited choice from a list of options, but is rather bounded by unique, subjective meanings inherent in every stress experience (Benner and Wrubel 1989).

In the current study, the cognitive, phenomenological, transactional framework allowed insight into the subjective, dynamic and reciprocal character of the stress that is experienced by both the nurses and the dying patient's relatives. The intrinsically stressful nature of the situation faced by relatives as they witnessed their loved one's worsening condition, while confronting their own impending loss, was vividly revealed in this study. The stress experienced by nurses who provide care during terminal illness, while simultaneously trying to respond to the multiple demands that the acute hospital setting presents, was also apparent. Moreover, the transactional character of the relationships that operated between relatives and nurses, and the factors within the ward environment that influenced both nurses' and relatives' perceptions of stress, emerged from the findings. The holistic and reflexive view of stress and coping as advanced by Benner and Wrubel (1989) substantially facilitated access to these insights.

In Chapter 2 two main coping modes were described: 'problem-focused' approaches that seek to remove or moderate stress at its source and 'emotion-focused' measures that aim to reduce the emotional impact of stress (Folkman 1984). It was clearly established that, although both modes tend to be used synchronously, their relative dominance will vary with the situation's potential for amelioration and with the personal, social and environmental coping resources available to counter the stress (Wrubel et al. 1981). The aptness of these theoretical concepts for exploring interpretations of the data are first considered in relation to the staff nurses' accounts and then in relation to the relatives' findings.

Stress and the staff nurses

The nurses' phase 1 data corroborates other evidence that providing support for relatives of dying patients generates feelings of stress in nurses (Ceslowitz 1989; E Hanson 1994). Phase 1 data from the current study also revealed a preponderance of emotion-focused strategies, with avoidance and distancing behaviour being commonly reported. There was scant evidence of problem-focused coping measures being applied by nurses during phase 1 of the study and a sense of powerlessness emerged from these data.

The nurses' phase 2 data differed from the phase 1 findings in several key ways. It appeared that nurses' appraisals of stress had altered over the course of the study, and it was notable that avoidance and distancing behaviour evident in the phase 1 accounts did not feature in the phase 2 data. Increased evidence emerged of the use of problem-solving behaviour, and frequent reports were offered of positive feelings of achievement resulting from the changes in their practice that many of the nurses had made. Just over half of the nurses reported deriving support from ward colleagues who had joined with them in their efforts to improve care in this area. Feelings of powerlessness and failure were much less evident, with almost every nurse reporting enhanced perceptions of self-efficacy and control. This finding lends support to Benner's claim that nursing's powerlessness is rooted in our beliefs about our own role rather than in the role itself (Benner and Wrubel 1989).

In contrast with the phase 1 findings, where the nurse–relative interface was revealed as somewhat tense and conflict ridden, the phase 2 accounts suggest that the closer relationships now established in most wards between nurses and relatives operated in a transactional and reflexive manner, thus generating mutual benefit. This finding supports evidence in the literature that the emotional energy that nurses require in order to continue to provide care in emotionally demanding situations (such as terminal care) often comes from the nurses' feelings of satisfaction in their work and from the positive feedback from those receiving care (Oberle and Davies 1992). These authors assert, and findings from the current study seem to confirm, that, when nurses are enabled to care in ways that are congruent with their personal beliefs and values, this has an empowering effect – thus acting as an important coping resource and a motivator for change (Oberle and Davies 1992). Benner and Wrubel (1989) similarly describe caring as an exchange of energy that can provide motivation and mutual support. They argue that, although connection and concern can set up personal involvement and mutual trust, 'non-caring' which they define as 'not being present' can cause patients (and relatives) to feel dehumanized, devalued, angry and fearful (Benner and Wrubel 1989).

This powerful image of a dynamic and reciprocal energy exchange taking place between caregivers and care recipients exemplifies the transactional character of stress and coping that was so clearly evident in both the nurses' and the relatives' accounts.

Discussion now focuses on the utility of the theoretical framework for illuminating the relatives' experiences.

Stress and the relatives

Relatives' experiences of stress in the days leading up to their loved one's death similarly reveal transactional and reciprocal qualities, although the range and type of coping strategies employed by relatives differed from the nurses in several respects. In both relatives' samples, stress was found to be primarily generated by their loved one's terminal illness and by their response to their own impending loss. As these situations were not amenable to amelioration, opportunities for problem-focused coping were limited. Consequently, both sets of relatives' data revealed a strong bias towards the use of emotion-focused or 'palliative' coping approaches (Folkman 1984).

Wrubel et al. (1981), the architects of the theoretical framework adopted for this study, suggest that, within every stressful encounter, factors within the situation, the environment and the individual will operate in a transactional and dynamic manner. These three major components of the stress experience are discussed below in relation to the relatives' experiences.

Factors within the situation

Wrubel et al. (1981) propose a number of potentially stressful elements within a situation which include (1) its uniqueness, (2) its duration and frequency, (3) its pervasiveness and (4) its potential for ambiguity (or uncertainty). Having to cope with terminal illness in a loved one was a situation faced by all of the relatives in the current study and, although each experience was unique, relatives reported common feelings of vulnerability, loss of control and helplessness related to their current situation.

Data from the current study reveal that when the illness had been of a long duration, e.g. spanning months or even years, and when the progression of the illness had been fluctuating and unpredictable in character, relatives' coping resources became undermined. The all-pervasive character of the relatives' situation was also highlighted in the data which revealed that every aspect of the relatives' current existence was permeated by their loved one's illness. Finally, relatives in the current study reported that, when they were unsure about what to expect and when they had unmet needs for information, their stress levels increased.

Of the situational factors described above, the need for information was the only factor amenable to manipulation within the current study. Comparing data from both samples of relatives confirms that, although stress associated with unmet needs for information represented a prominent feature in the phase 1 accounts, all but two relatives in phase 2 reported satisfaction with the information they received from nurses. However, just over a third of the phase 2 relatives reported experiencing stress as a result of difficulties in gaining access to, and getting information from, medical staff.

Factors within the environment

Environmental influences were particularly relevant as potential stressors because data from the current study suggest that the intimidating nature of the acute hospital environment can have the effect of limiting relatives' coping options. Phase 2 data from the current study, and from the literature (Wros 1993), suggest that relatives' coping resources were supported by interventions that modified aspects of the hospital environment, and that made the ward less threatening and more welcoming and comfortable for the family. The phase 2 data also reveal the coping benefits that result when relatives are able to be with their dying loved one in a quiet, private setting and when the attending family have access to facilities for rest and refreshment.

Other factors to emerge within the ward environment relate to relationships between relatives and nurses. Data from both relatives and nurses, in both phases of the study, indicate that changes in the nature of these relationships occurred. In all but one of the study wards, closer and more relaxed relationships were reported to be operating between nurses and relatives during the post-intervention period of the study, and the data indicated that this yielded reciprocal coping benefits. The transactional properties of coping are supported by Nugent (1988) who asserts that supportive social relationships appear to be central to most coping activity, and that coping effectiveness tends to be highly dependent on the influence of others.

Factors within the individual

Approaches to stress based on trait theories tend to reify desirable dispositions and equate these with such constructs as 'good copers'. In contrast, transactional theories recognize that within every stressful encounter an individual's appraisal of threat can vary, as can their judgements about their own self-efficacy and their access to coping support.

Data from both samples of relatives revealed heavy reliance on psychological defence mechanisms such as hope and denial. The theoretical framework offered a fruitful vehicle for seeking deeper insights into the complex and fluctuating nature of these states. The data suggest that, for close relatives of dying patients, hope and denial operated as buffers against the stress caused by the loved one's imminent death. As imminent loss of a loved one was a situation common to both samples, and as this situation was not amenable to manipulation, no marked differences emerged between the pre- and post-intervention relatives' samples in the range and frequency of use of these strategies.

Insights gained into hope and denial, and particularly into their fluctuating and reciprocal qualities, developed over the course of the study and deepened significantly during interpretation of the phase 2 relatives' data. These heightened perceptions were derived from several sources which included the multiple perspectives offered by a larger body of relatives' data, the maturing skills of the interpreter and insights gained from the literature (Owen 1989; Scanlon 1989; Herth 1990; Perakyla 1991; Herth 1993).

The cognitive, phenomenological, transactional model of stress and coping proved to be a useful and illuminating framework for interpreting and reporting data from both nurses and relatives, and for illustrating the reflexive and dynamic influences that operate between the relatives and nurses in a hospital environment, and in particular within the situational context of terminal illness. Stress and coping represented enduring and pervasive themes throughout the entire investigation and were omnipresent in the literature that has been consulted in the course of this study.

However, a theoretical framework is useful as a tool for understanding and as a guide to practice only if it can illuminate complex processes and assist in explicating these in a coherent way. The design of the current study included two discrete phases separated by an extended and complex intervention, and incorporated three different samples and a range of data-gathering approaches including interview data and evaluation data from the quality assurance standards and from the workshop. In the light of this complexity, it was judged important to have a coherent, holistic and yet reflexive analytical framework running through the entire investigation, which would permit comparisons to be drawn between pre- and post-intervention data and which would enable associations between the data sets to emerge when interpreting the findings. The cognitive, phenomenological, transactional model of stress and coping served these needs very well.

Nevertheless, controversy abounds as to how central extant theory should be in an investigation or indeed whether such an approach can ever be justified within the interpretative paradigm. Although some committed phenomenologists maintain that the voice of the data should be heard to speak alone and without recourse to theory as a filter through which to view a phenomenon, others would dispute the need to ban extant theory from interpretation, advocating rather that theoretical interpretation be seen as a final, enhancing step in the interpretative process (Kvale 1983; Benner and Wrubel 1989; Sandelowski 1993a).

It has also been cogently argued that theory can legitimately enter and leave (and indeed re-enter) a study at different points in the investigation (Sandelowski 1993a). Theory can also be applied centrally or peripherally within an investigation, with the peripheral use of theory being rather like 'brushstroking the theory in to aid interpretation' (Sandelowski 1993a). Within the current study theoretical interpretations were applied in precisely that way because it was only at the final stage in the analysis process that, in an effort to further elucidate insights or to confirm associations that had emerged from the data, links with theory were made.

Review of the intervention

In the early stages of the study, an evaluation design was selected because the intention was to evaluate an educational intervention in the form of a learning package. This decision was later reviewed in the light of findings from the pilot study data, confirmed in the literature, that the major concerns of both nurses and relatives related to aspects of communication. This suggested that the changes that might be required were likely to have an attitudinal component.

The literature offers good evidence that communication and relationship issues are most effectively dealt with by using experiential learning approaches (Wilkinson 1991; Candlin 1992; Baynton-Lees 1993). Moreover, it has also been reported in Chapter 6 that ownership of, and hence commitment to, a change initiative is enhanced when those required to implement change also design the change strategy (Harvey 1994; Gibson 1995). For these reasons, a quality assurance framework using ward-based clinical standards was selected as the mechanism for implementing the changes in practice.

In the light of these factors, the intervention approach was revised to incorporate a 2-day workshop that would facilitate the feedback of the phase 1 research data and the development of research-based quality assurance standards and also provide a suitable climate for an experiential learning approach for addressing communication issues. It should be acknowledged that, despite the potential advantages and utility of standard setting as a change strategy, this intervention approach was not selected without some reservation.

Philosophical tensions in standard setting

Standards have long been heralded as the hallmarks of a profession because they serve the joint goals of self-regulation and the promotion of quality for the consumer (Lang and Wessel Krejci 1991). Nursing faces particular problems in articulating its unique and holistic contribution to care within a health-care system with resource-driven pressures to produce measurable outcomes. This concern is particularly salient in the area of standard setting which, by itemizing and decontextualizing care, risks losing the very essence of holism in nursing. Although entities such as care, compassion and presence are fundamental to the quality of care, as experienced by the consumer, they do not easily lend themselves well to techniques of measurement or calibration often demanded when evaluating standards. This dissonance was acknowledged some 15 years ago when it was noted that, as human beings need *both* quantifiable and unquantifiable care, it is clearly necessary to articulate a world view of nursing that will reflect both its human paradigm and the one that is still quantifiable (Paulen 1980).

Nursing is one of the few disciplines to have successfully merged the traditional sciences with the art of caring. It should therefore be possible to resolve the reductionism–holism tension presented by standard setting by combining traditional objective criteria, when evaluating standards, with the subjective perspectives of those who receive and those who provide care (Lang and Wessel Krejci 1991). This precisely represents the approach to standard setting and evaluation adopted in the current study, and it underscores the point that standards and holism need not be philosophically incompatible. Indeed, within the current study the motivating force that drove the standard-setting initiative forward was the nurses' desire to provide care within a more humanistic and holistic framework.

However, a practical yet unforeseen difficulty with employing a standard-setting approach was that the scope of attempted change, and the consultation and negotiations that were required, meant that to bring the standards to the stage of implementation took between 6 and 8 months and involved much effort from all concerned.

As the results of these efforts have already been reported from the subjective perspectives of the relatives (Chapter 7) and the nurses (Chapter 8), discussion focuses on some issues that influenced the change process in the study wards.

Analysis of change

Lewin's useful concept of 'Force Field Analysis' facilitates analysis of the driving forces that facilitate change and restraining forces that inhibit change within most planned change initiatives (Bennis et al. 1985; Tiffany et al. 1994). In the current study, the crucial driving force came from the staff nurses who, in their change agent capacity, represented the 'leverage point' that provided the momentum for change. In the researcher's judgement, changes were most evident in those wards where the change agents were experienced, charismatic, opinion leaders who could carry their ward teams along with them. Conversely, less confident and less affiliated nurses seemed to experience more difficulty in driving the change initiative forward. The influence of the change agent's personality on the success of a change initiative has been widely reported in the literature, where the benefits of a support network for the change agent are also emphasized (Stevenson 1990).

The post-workshop evaluation data and the nurses' phase 2 interview data revealed that the staff nurses' main support came from the researcher, their 'partner' change agent in the ward and their ward colleagues. The data also indicated that, in wards where collaborative relationships operated between medical and nursing staff, the overall magnitude of change seemed to be greater. Conversely, there was evidence to suggest that change was difficult to achieve in wards with a hierarchical management style and where the balance of professional power rested mainly with the medical staff. The implications that this climate has for autonomy and advocacy in nursing are reported in the literature (Greenwood 1994) and were also evident in the current study.

Barriers to change

An illustrative summary of the barriers to change that can operate within a planned change initiative in the hospital setting, and which may ultimately lead to complete failure of uptake of change, is given below. This takes the form of an analysis of factors evident within the single ward where the change initiative was unsuccessful.

Analysis of failed change

Impressions about the staff nurse/change agent were formed over an 18-month period and revealed her to be a somewhat tense person who seemed to be perpetually harassed. Her 'study partner' staff nurse had moved to another ward during the pre-intervention period and her efforts to recruit a replacement partner from the ward team were unsuccessful. Consequently, she lacked the peer support found to be so important to the other nurses. She also reported very 'patchy' support from the ward team and no support at all from her nurse manager. To compound these difficulties, the ward sister changed during the course of the study. Finally, and crucially, a striking feature of this ward was the professional hierarchy that operated within the care 'team'. Indeed, during a conversation about the study, the researcher was firmly informed by the senior consultant in this ward that 'nurses have neither the right nor the authority to make changes in hospitals'. It was therefore not surprising that in such a climate the change initiative foundered and the standard, although written, was never implemented.

While acknowledging that the situation analysed above represents a single and perhaps extreme example of barriers to change, some degree of unresolved difficulty was reported in most wards in the area of interprofessional communication and in the area of relatives' access to information from medical staff. It is possible that a change initiative that had adopted an interdisciplinary approach might have elicited greater collaboration and commitment from the medical staff.

The planned change approach used in this study enabled staff in the wards to design, implement and evaluate their own change strategy. Although it would have been surprising if there had been uniform success and acceptance of the initiative in every ward, the method adopted offered the best chance of initiating a change process and of sustaining the energy needed to maintain it.

The stability of change

It has been revealed in the literature that reinforcement and feed-back to the target group can help to sustain the momentum of change and maintain the stability of change (Swansburg 1993). In the current study, feedback was provided mainly by the researcher's regular contact with the nurses. Also helpful was the team spirit, soli-darity and healthy competition that developed between members of the study team in different wards and between nurses in both hospi-tals. Reinforcement was also provided by the nurses' attendance at conferences and study days, where they heard their work reported and where one of the staff nurses also presented a paper on her study activities.

A final study day was also conducted to allow the staff nurses to hear the feedback from the phase 2 findings and to enable them to share their experiences, triumphs and frustrations with other members of the study team. The final study day also provided a forum where the nurses could discuss their future plans for develop-ments in the provision of family-centred care.

Major insights gained from the study

Several important insights were gained from this study and these were substantially facilitated by the dual perspectives offered by the nurses and the relatives. The most striking of insights relate to the reflexive character of the stress that is experienced by relatives of dying patients in hospital and the nurses who provide care, and the transactional nature of their coping responses. The data also reveal that support strategies often yield reciprocal benefits, in that measures taken to support relatives were also commonly found to support the nurses and to reduce their levels of stress. This was most powerfully revealed in relation to nurse–relative communication, where nurses' approach strategies to the family changed, and in rela-tion to the provision of facilities for relatives.

The pre-intervention data highlighted the nature of the barriers that exist to effective nurse–relative communication. These barriers were found to exist at the point of contact and the phase 1 data offered evidence of the discomfort that both relatives and nurses experience when approaching each other.

It was revealed in Chapter 5 that the phase 1 relatives commonly felt inhibited about approaching nurses whom they generally perceived to be too busy to be interrupted. A frequently expressed concern of relatives was that they did not want to be seen as a 'nuisance' by disturbing busy nurses. Many relatives also reported not knowing whom they should approach and when; consequently, relatives reported unmet needs for information and support.

The nurses' discomfort about approaching relatives also stemmed from several sources. The phase 1 data suggest that the nurses' perceptions of relatives' high expectations had an intimidating effect and the anticipation of failure that this generated caused them to avoid initiating contact with relatives in the ward. The data also suggest that nurses felt further constrained by lack of privacy when communicating with relatives, lack of knowledge about the relatives' current awareness of their loved ones' prognosis and lack of confidence in their own communication skills. The phase 1 data also confirm that the nurses experience stress when dealing with relatives and that nurses also had significant unmet needs for support.

The effect of the intervention was to dismantle some of these barriers and to do so in quite simple but fundamental ways. When the relatives' feelings and experiences were illuminated through the phase 1 data and were presented to the nurses, this had a truly galvanizing effect. The feedback of the phase 1 data, and the experiential workshop that followed, caused the nurses to re-evaluate their communication skills and to reassess their own potential to change aspects of the environment of care and their own practice. These perceptual shifts enabled reappraisals to be made of the level of threat that this aspect of care presented, as a result of which new possibilities for coping emerged and the nurses' level of personal comfort in their role increased. From this new world view, the nurses' approach strategies to relatives changed, nurse–relative dialogue flourished and relationships with the family were established. The data from *both* relatives and nurses reveal that this resulted in a reduction in the nurses' use of distancing and avoidance tactics, and in a reciprocal reduction in the level of stress reported by both relatives and nurses.

The crucial importance of providing a private area where relatives could rest and receive information and support from staff was also revealed in both the nurses' and the relatives' accounts. There was evidence to suggest that such a facility not only supports the relatives during an emotionally intense experience, but also acts as a potent coping resource for nurses. When nurses were able to offer such amenities they reported a reduction in their own subjective experience of stress, which in turn resulted in reduced use of distancing behaviour and in enhanced communication.

A powerful insight from this study was therefore that a relatives' room represents a crucial coping resource for both relatives and staff, and it has significant potential to enhance the quality of care during terminal illness. Furthermore, when the crucial areas of communication and facilities were improved and nurses felt able to deliver high-quality care, the positive feedback that this generated provided the impetus needed to implement improvements in other areas.

Another compelling message in the data relates to the dynamic characteristics of denial and hope. The data strongly suggested that denial, often regarded as a rather negative concept, operates as an important coping strategy that most individuals employ in fluctuating measure and with considerable insight in the time leading up to the death of a loved one. Also, the complexity of hope, and its reflexive relationship to denial, so poignantly revealed in the current study, has also been reported in the literature (Scanlon 1989; Perakyla 1991; Janes 1992; Herth 1993; Shea and Kendrick 1995).

It is crucial that nurses recognize that for the patient and close family openly to acknowledge the imminence of death can require a shift in emotional orientation within the relationship, which can be of such magnitude and profound significance, that, for some, it will represent a step quite beyond contemplation. For such families, although there might be tacit acknowledgement of the reality of death, pretence continues to the end.

For others, as described in the second paradigm (see pages 201–203), open disclosure of the prognosis is preferred. When this point is reached, hope of recovery is finally dismantled, denial is shelved, and the reality of the forthcoming death is confronted openly by the patient and family. In such situations nurses must be acutely sensitive to the needs of a grieving patient and family, with all of the implications that this has for their needs for privacy, support and comfort.

Limitations of the study

A number of limitations must be acknowledged in a study of this nature. First, the single interview approach, which was used with a large majority of the relatives, clearly could offer only a snapshot of what must be a dynamic experience during which needs and concerns might change over time. However, given the nature of the situation, it was not possible to incorporate repeat interviews with relatives because in most cases their loved one died within a week of the interview.

Furthermore, the nature of the situation made it necessary for separate samples of relatives to be recruited for the phase 1 and the phase 2 interviews. Although both relatives' samples were broadly comparable in terms of age and relationship to the patient, drawing comparisons in this way is always problematic. Potential sampling bias must also be accepted because it is possible that those relatives approached by the nurses might not have been wholly representative. It should be stated, however, that this seems unlikely because evidence from the literature offers no reason to suppose that the relatives included in this study's samples were in any way unrepresentative.

Also, as this study sought to achieve attitudinal change, and as it involved an extended researcher–participant relationship within a complex change process, an attitude of distance on the part of the researcher would have been not just inappropriate but also undesirable. The centrality of the researcher–participant relationship to the action research approach that was ultimately employed, and the reflexive nature of the relationships that operated within the study, demanded a commitment to self-scrutiny and a willingness to respond, develop and change as the investigation unfolded.

Finally, although the analysis approach adopted in this study provided revealing insights that illuminated the lived experiences and concerns of both relatives and nurses, 'pure' phenomenologists could argue persuasively that the depth of interpretation might have been limited by the very large volume of data that was generated by 80 interviews.

Applicability of the findings

Insights that have emerged from this study have wide applicability to practice because they have the potential to deepen understanding and heighten awareness of a range of issues that are salient for relatives of dying patients in hospital wards and for the nurses who provide their care.

It has already been reported in Chapter 4 that the deepest level of hermeneutic interpretation occurs when participants respond to the research data by engaging in corrective action (Kvale 1983). It was similarly suggested that a study can claim 'catalytic authenticity' if the research findings motivate the reader to take action and that it has 'tactical authenticity' when the work empowers practitioners to bring about positive change (Guba and Lincoln 1994).

It was precisely this type of empowerment that was generated by the phase 1 interview data and resulted in the staff nurses engaging in dynamic and collaborative action aimed at changing both their practice and the environment of care. By combined processes of diffusion and dissemination, news of the study findings, and of the changes that the nurses in the study wards had made, spread to other wards, other hospitals and indeed to several other countries. The findings from this study therefore have wide applicability both within hospital practice and in other care settings within the UK and elsewhere.

The findings confirm the reciprocal benefits that can be accrued by improving the facilities provided for relatives of dying patients, and by implementing simple but crucial changes in communication patterns with families. The findings also underscore the benefits of providing opportunities for professional education and support in this area.

Conclusions

Although care at home represents a desirable option for some dying patients and their families, for others problems in achieving adequate symptom control, the onset of acute medical crisis or severe caregiver stress can all lead to hospital admission in the weeks or days leading up to the patient's death. Caring for dying patients and their families therefore remains a significant aspect of acute hospital nursing practice.

This study has confirmed that, by the time relatives have relinquished care of their dying loved one, they have already experienced significant stress and this stress is often compounded by feelings of guilt associated with the final admission. The support needs of such relatives are therefore considerable.

When the dying patient's relatives remain in the ward for long periods of time, staff can face a range of difficulties as they seek to accommodate and relate to the family. The phase 1 data revealed that, in the emotionally charged situation of terminal illness, relationships between nurses and relatives could be somewhat uneasy and conflict ridden. This was exposed in the liberal use of 'war metaphors' in the nurses' phase 1 data.

The phase 2 data offered a striking contrast. Nurses had seemingly lowered their guard and moved in closer to establish an emotional connection with the family. The phase 2 relatives commonly described the ward atmosphere as friendly and relaxed and the facilities some wards now offer for relatives' comfort were frequently praised. The reciprocal benefits of these altered relationships, and of the improved facilities, offered a compelling message in the phase 2 data.

Issues for nurses

The nurses' phase 1 data highlighted difficulties nurses faced in the acute setting, where they reported stress caused by multiple demands and competing priorities. Although many claimed to prefer to practise within a holistic framework, the pace and level of activity in the ward seemed to hinder their efforts. Nurses also felt restricted in wards that lacked facilities for relatives and in practice settings where professional hierarchies featured strongly.

Attitudinal issues separate from, yet intrinsically linked to, the above factors also surfaced. The phase 1 data confirmed a tendency to view the patient as the sole focus of care. The shift that occurred in many study wards to a more holistic and family-oriented approach to terminal care markedly altered this situation. From this new perspective, the dying patient's family became intrinsic to, rather than adjuncts of, the care. More spontaneous interactions between nurses and relatives were established and a concern for and involvement in the provision of family support developed.

A serendipitous outcome was that in connecting emotionally with the family the nurses' own reported stress levels decreased.

Recommendations

To offer a series of prescriptive recommendations based on the findings of this study would not be congruent with its overall ethos, which has aimed to be practice based, facilitative and inductive in orientation.

This research study incorporated a ward-based change agent approach to design, implement and monitor planned changes in practice. Crucial to the success of the change initiative was that those involved in bringing the changes about also designed the change strategy. In this study the change strategy involved quality assurance standards.

Research

Insights gained from this study came from nurses and relatives in acute hospital wards in two city hospitals. It might therefore be useful to undertake a replication of this research in other acute hospitals because statistical data confirm that most patients die in this setting. In particular it may be useful to repeat the approach using fewer wards and more staff in each ward, e.g. identifying two, or at most three, wards in which terminal care is a regular feature, and involving the whole ward team in the change process, might yield interesting insights into the dynamics of change.

The study design could also be modified to research relatives' support in different institutional and non-institutional terminal care settings. Also dissemination of the research-based standards could be undertaken to monitor their use in other wards, possibly using different levels of support to determine how best to achieve changes in practice. Issues of ownership would, however, have to be considered when implementing such initiatives.

This study also highlighted unresolved issues relating to interprofessional communication. Multiprofessional initiatives that encourage collaborative working in this area are therefore recommended. The study design used in this research could be modified to incorporate the medical staff into the change initiative. Another approach might be to set up quality circles because these favour collaborative practice. Multidisciplinary audit tools could be developed based on the findings of the current study. Suggested questions for inclusion in a research-based audit tool are included as Appendix 2. Other key concepts to emerge from this research include the complex and reciprocal character of hope and denial. The implications that these coping strategies have for patients, relatives and in particular professional carers within the context of terminal care merit further study.

Practice

This study confirms the supportive benefits for both relatives and staff of providing a comfortable, private area where the dying patient's close family can rest and where they can receive information and support from staff. Findings from this research have also revealed the benefits of providing facilities for rest and comfort when relatives remain at their loved one's bedside overnight. The findings highlighted the value of a folding bed for this purpose. The provision of a folding bed, or at the very least a recliner chair and blankets and a pillow, for the overnight comfort of relatives is therefore recommended.

The study findings have also revealed that, although communication with this group is not easy, strategies can be developed to create a more comfortable interface between relatives and nurses. Such strategies depend heavily on enhancing the nurses' feelings of comfort during interactions with the family. It was convincingly, and repeatedly, reported in this study that nurses' stress is reduced when they can communicate with the family within a setting that meets the privacy needs of both the relatives and the nurse. Measures to improve facilities for the comfort and privacy of the dying patient's relatives in hospital are therefore urgently recommended.

Education

Nurses require opportunities to increase their competence and confidence in the area of communication. This study has revealed substantial evidence of unmet needs for access to courses or study days that deal with interpersonal issues within the context of terminal illness. Educational initiatives such as experiential learning workshops are recommended, where nurses can share concerns and can refine their communication skills in a non-threatening setting. This recommendation is also convincingly supported in the research literature (Wilkinson 1991; Corner and Wilson-Barnett 1992).

The findings from this research confirm the transactional nature of the stress that is experienced by both relatives of dying patients and the nurses who provide terminal care in hospitals. It has been established that, although the source of that stress was not amenable to amelioration, it was possible to support and augment the coping resources of both relatives and nurses by modifying the physical environment and enhancing the emotional climate of care.

> Nurses do not cure stress but they can help people to survive it by establishing a healing relationship and by helping them to mobilize their emotional and spiritual resources.
>
> (Benner and Wrubel 1989, p. 62)

Appendix 1
Standard of nursing care

Standard of nursing care

Standard reference: REN 3 S
Topic: Terminal Nursing Care
Sub Topic: Care of Relatives
Care Group: Relatives of terminally ill patients
Local Reference:

Index Code:
Review Standard by:
Signature Senior Nurse: ....
Signature Director of Nursing: ....
Date of Validation: ....

Directorate:
Standard Statement: Relatives/significant others of terminally ill patients will be offered the maximum physical, psychological and spiritual support during the terminal stages of the patient's illness

Structure	Process	Outcome
Facilities for comfort and privacy	The nurse will undertake to:	O.1 relatives have access to a designated room within which their needs for privacy and support can be met
The Unit can offer	P.1 maintain the room and equipment in a clean, comfortable condition	
S.1 a private room designed specifically for relatives' use	P.2 inform relatives of their access to:	O.2 all members of the multidisciplinary team are aware of the range of facilities in the unit and will utilize these as required
S.2 provision of furniture to enable relatives to rest during the day and night in comfort and privacy	• the relatives' room • facilities for rest during the day and night • facilities for making tea and coffee	O.3 relatives of dying patients can obtain rest, sleep and refreshments in a private area which is close to the patient
S.3 facilities for making refreshments		
S.4 a reclining chair or z-bed for relatives who wish to stay overnight at the bedside	P.4 provide a reclining chair for relatives who wish to stay overnight at the bedside	O.4 relatives who wish to stay overnight can rest in a recliner chair
S.5a access to a phone, shops and facilities for obtaining meals in the canteen	P.5a offer relatives directions to the shops, telephone and the hospital canteen	O.5 relatives know the layout of the hospital and can locate:
S.5b access to toilet and washing machine facilities	P.5b direct relatives to toilets and washing facilities	• telephone and shops • the hospital canteen • toilet and washing facilities

Structure	Process	Outcome
Staff/relative communication	P.6 relatives are made comfortable in the relatives' room prior to receiving information or having discussions with members of the care team	O.6 relatives receive information and counselling within a private, appropriate setting
S.6 a private area is available where members of the staff and care team can provide information/offer counselling to relatives		
S.7 agreed procedures exist to enable a nurse to be present when the relatives receive new information	P.7 in nursing 7 medical staff communicate prior to meetings, to enable a nurse to be present when new information is given to relatives	O.7 both medical and nursing staff are fully aware of relatives' current knowledge and acceptance of the prognosis and treatment
S.8 a record of multidisciplinary referrals and outcomes is available	P.8 the nurse will record multidisciplinary meetings, referrals and outcomes in the nursing notes	O.8 staff involved in family support have access to a current record of referrals and outcomes
Social and spiritual support	P.9 the nurse will, in discussions with relatives, establish their need for access to the Social Worker and arrange appointments as required	O.9 relatives are able to express their socio-economic needs and to have support and advice from a Social Worker
S.9 a Social Worker is available to relatives who need specific help and advice		
an information folder is available at the nurses' station which contains —	P.10 the nurse will maintain and update the list of spiritual advisors and will make this information available to relatives	O.10 relatives receive spiritual support in accordance with their wishes and needs
S.10 a list of contact numbers for spiritual advisors		O.11 relatives can travel to the hospital with the minimum delay and inconvenience
S.11 information about transport i.e bus and train timetables and taxi phone numbers	P.11 the nurse will offer information about transport times and phone numbers and will update this information as required	O.12 nursing staff are aware of the policies and procedures to follow to enable them to support relatives at the time of death

(Continued)

Structure	Process	Outcome
Support and information around the time of death	P.12 the nurse will maintain and update the GGHB guidelines file and ensure that ward nursing staff are aware of its location	O.13 newly bereaved relatives are able to express their grief within a sensitive private setting and are offered comfort, support and information
S.12 the information folder contains guidelines which include policy and procedures and details the responsibilites of nursing staff around the time of death	P.13 following the patient's death the nurse will take the family to the relatives' room and will • offer comfort, sympathy • provide verbal guidance about what the relatives need to do following the death • provide written guidance if needed	O.14 relatives are clear about what they need to do following the patient's death
S.13 an information booklet is available to newly bereaved relatives		
S.14 a nurse known to the family will be available to offer comfort, support and information around the time of death	P.14 the nurse will use sensitive questioning to check that the relatives have understood the information which has been given	

Evaluation of clinical standard

Use a fresh sheet with each family   Standard applied to the family of –

Topic   <u>Terminal Nursing Care</u>   Sub Topic   Care of relatives

<u>Standard Statement:</u>   Relatives/significant others of terminally ill patients will be offered the maximum physical, psychological and spiritual support during the terminal stages of the patient's illness

Care Group   Relatives of terminally ill patients in   Assessed by ....

S/P/O No.	Criteria (worded in question form)	Measured by	Achieved Yes No	Date	Signed	Comments
	<u>Is the unit able to offer?</u>					
S.1	a clean private area for the use of relatives	observing				
S.2	facilities for rest and sleep	"				
S.3	access to refreshments	"				
	<u>Is the following information available within the unit?</u>					
S.10	• an update of religious advisors	asking and records				
S.11	• Information about transport	asking				
S.12	• a list of guidelines including policy, detailing the responsibilities of the nurse following the patient's death	observing and asking				
O.6	did relatives receive information and counselling within a private sensitive setting?	observing and records				
P.7	were nurses present at meetings when information was being relayed to relatives?	"				
O.8	does a record exist of meetings, referrals and their outcomes?	"				
O.13	were relatives able to express their grief and offered support and information within a private non-clinical setting?	"				
P.14	on sensitive questioning – were relatives clear about what they needed to do following the death of the patient?	asking				

Appendix 2
Proposed framework for ward audit

Support for the dying patient's family in hospital

Relatives' communication with nursing staff

- Do nursing staff initiate and then regularly maintain contact with relatives for communication and emotional support?
- Is a private area available where relatives can receive information and support?
- Do relatives have access to a named nurse during each duty span?
- Do relatives receive a daily update from nurses on the condition and care of their loved one?

Relatives' communication with medical staff

- Are relatives able to meet with a member of the medical staff for information and advice and are such meetings either (a) spontaneously offered or (b) arranged within 24 hours of the relatives' request?

Facilities for privacy, comfort and rest

- Are dying patients and their relatives cared for in a single room if desired?
- Is there an area for relatives to have periods of rest away from the bedside?
- When staying overnight at the bedside are facilities such as a folding bed or recliner chair and blankets offered to enable relatives to rest?
- Are regular refreshments provided or made available?
- Do relatives have convenient access to toilet and washing facilities?

Social and spiritual support

• Where appropriate are relatives referred to the hospital social worker for financial or other advice?
• Around the time of the patient's death;-
Are relatives comforted within a private setting by a member of staff who is known to the family?
Is information about spiritual advisors and death registration procedures provided if this is required?
Are the patient's belongings returned in a sensitive appropriate manner?

Interprofessional communication

To facilitate coordinated multidisciplinary family support;

• Do measures/procedures exist to ensure that nurses are made aware of the family's knowledge about and acceptance of the prognosis?
• Is a nurse present when relatives receive information about their loved one's prognosis?
• Are referrals and meetings with other team members of the care team (and their outcomes) recorded and accessible to nursing staff?
• Are members of the care team given opportunities to attend courses or study days on care of the dying and bereaved and on aspects of communication and counselling?

References

Akinsanya J (1994). Making research useful to the practising nurse. *Journal of Advanced Nursing* **19**(1): 174–9.

Alexander DA (1990). Stressors and difficulties in dealing with the terminal patient. *Journal of Palliative Care* **6**(3): 28–33.

Altheide DL, Johnson JM (1994). Criteria for assessing interpretive validity in qualitative research. In: *Handbook of Qualitative Research*, Denzin N, Lincoln Y, eds. Thousand Oaks, CA: Sage Publications Inc.: Chapter 30.

Anstey S (1993). Care in acute hospital units. *Nursing Standard* **7**(19): 51.

Antonovsky A (1987). *Unravelling the mystery of health; How people manage stress and stay well.* California, CA: Jossey-Bass Inc.

Aranda S (1995). Conducting research with the dying: ethical considerations and experience. *International Journal of Palliative Nursing* **1**(1): 41–7.

Archbold P (1986). Ethical issues in qualitative research. In: *From Practice to Grounded Theory: Qualitative research in nursing*, Chenitz WC, Swanson JM, eds. Menlo Park, CA: Addison-Wesley, pp. 155–63.

Armitage P, Burnard P (1991). Mentors or preceptors? Narrowing the theory–practice gap. *Nurse Education Today* **11**: 225–9.

Atwood J, Hinds P (1986). Heuristic heresy: application of reliability and validity criteria to products of grounded theory. *Western Journal of Nursing Research* **8**: 152–4.

Bacon D (1993). Struggle and reward: working with staff under pressure. *Journal of the Royal Society of Medicine* **86**: 427–8.

Baglioni AJ, Cooper CL, Hingley P (1990). Job stress, mental health and job satisfaction among UK senior nurses. *Stress Medicine* **6**(1): 9–20.

Bailley R, Clarke M (1989). *Stress and Coping in Nursing*. London: Chapman & Hall.

Baker C, Wuest J, Noeranger Stern P (1992). Method slurring; the grounded theory/phenomenology example. *Journal of Advanced Nursing* **17**: 1355–60.

Bakhurst D (1992). Debate – on lying and deceiving. *Journal of Medical Ethics* **18**: 63–6.

Basset C (1992). The integration of research in the clinical setting: obstacles and solutions. A review of literature. *Nursing Practice* **6**(1): 4–8.

Baynton-Lees D (1993). Setting the scene for experiential learning. *Nursing Standard* **7**(36): 28–30.

Beauchamp T, Childress JF (1983). *Principles of Bio-Medical Ethics*. Oxford: Oxford University Press.

Benner P (1983). Uncovering the knowledge embedded in clinical practice. *Image* **15**(2): 36–41.

Benner P (1985). Quality of life: A phenomenological perspective on explanation, prediction and understanding in nursing science. *Advances in Nursing Science* **8**(11): 1–14.

Benner P, ed. (1994). *Interpretive Phenomenology; Embodiment, Caring and Ethics in Health and Illness*. Thousand Oaks, CA: Sage Publications.

Benner P, Wrubel J (1988). Caring comes first. *American Journal of Nursing* **88**: 1072–5.

Benner PE, Wrubel J (1989). *The Primacy of Caring: Stress and coping in health and illness*. Menlo Park, CA: Addison-Wesley Publishing Co.

Bennis W, Benne K, Chin R, eds (1985). *The Planning of Change*. New York: Holt, Rhinehart & Winston.

Benoliel JQ, McCorkle R, Georgiadou F, Denton T, Spitzer A (1990). Measurement of stress in clinical nursing. *Cancer Nursing* **13**: 221–8.

Bhola HS (1994). The CLER Model: thinking through change. *Nursing Management* **25**(5): 59–63.

Birch J (1979). The anxious learners. *Nursing Mirror* Feb 17th: 17–24.

Blumer H (1969). *Symbolic Interactionism: Perspective and method*. Englewood Cliffs, NJ: Prentice Hall.

Bolton Health Council (1986). *Care of the Dying in Bolton: Report on a survey of 51 bereaved relatives of cancer patients*. Bolton Community Health Council,.

Bowers L (1992) Ethnomethodology I: an approach to nursing research. Part I. *International Journal of Nursing Studies* **29**(1): 59–67.

Bowling A (1991). Health care research methods – Part 1. *Nursing Standard* **5**(48): 34–7.

Broome A (1990). *Managing Change*. London: Macmillan.

Buchan J (1995). Nurses' estimations of patients' prognoses in the last days of life. *International Journal of Palliative Nursing* **1**(1): 12–16.

Burns N, Grove S (1993). *The Practice of Nursing Research: Conduct, critique and utilization*. Philadelphia, PA: WB Saunders Co.

Candlin S (1992). Communication for nurses; implications for nurse education. *Nurse Education Today* **12**: 445–51.

Cartwright A (1991). Changes in life and care in the year before death 1969–1987. *Journal of Public Health Medicine* **13**(2).

Cartwright A, Hockey L, Anderson JL (1973). *Life before Death*. London: Routledge & Keegan Paul Ltd.

Ceslowitz SB (1989). Burnout and coping strategies among hospital staff nurses. *Journal of Advanced Nursing* **14**: 553–7.

Cheddel A (1991). Nursing standards are standard. *Nursing Standard* **5**(41): 54–5.

Cherniss C (1980). *Staff Burnout: Job stress in the human services*. London: Sage Publications Inc.

Chodil JJ, Dulaney PE (1984). Continuing education on dying and death – does participation in a workshop on dying and death decrease the nurses' death anxiety? *Journal of Continuing Education in Nursing* **15**(1): 5–8.

Clarke J (1991). Moral dilemmas in nursing research. *Nursing Practice* **4**(4): 22–5.

Clarke JB, Wheeler SJ (1992). A view of the phenomenon of caring in nursing practice. *Journal of Advanced Nursing* **17**: 1283–90.

Clarke M (1984). Stress and coping: constructs for nursing. *Journal of Advanced Nursing* **9**: 3–13.

Cole A (1992). High anxiety. *Nursing Times* **88**(12): 26–31.

Connors D (1988). A continuum of researcher–participant relationships; An analysis and critique. *Advances in Nursing Science* **10**(4): 32–42.

Corner J (1991a). Cancer nursing research. *Nursing Times* **87**(37): 42–4.

Corner J (1991b). In search of more complete answers to research questions. Quantitative versus qualitative research methods: is there a way forward? *Journal of Advanced Nursing* **16**: 718–27.

Corner J, Wilson-Barnett J (1992). The newly registered nurse and the cancer patient: an educational evaluation. *International Journal of Nursing Studies* **29**: 177–90.

Crowley SA, Wollner IS (1987). Collaborative practice: A tool for change. *Oncology Nursing Forum* **14**(4): 59–63.

Darbyshire P (1992). Parenting in public: A study of the experience of parents who live in with their hospitalised child, and of their relationship with paediatric nurses. Unpublished thesis, University of Edinburgh.

Davies B (1990). Families in supportive care – Part 1 : The transition of fading away: The nature of the transition. *Journal of Palliative Care* **6**(3): 12–30.

Davies B, Oberle K (1990). Dimensions of the supportive role of the nurse in palliative care. *Oncology Nursing Forum* **17**(1): 87–94.

Davies B, Reimer J, Martens N (1994). Family functioning and its implications for palliative care. *Journal of Palliative Care* **10**(1): 29–36.

Degner LF, Gow CM (1988a). Evaluations of death education in nursing: a critical review. *Cancer Nursing* **11**: 151–9.

Degner LF, Gow CM (1988b). Preparing nurses for care of the dying: A longitudinal study. *Cancer Nursing* **11**: 160–9.

Dewe P (1987). Identifying the causes of nurses' stress: a survey of New Zealand nurses. *Work and Stress* **1**(1): 15–34.

Dicks B (1990). Palliative care for cancer patients. *Nursing Standard* **4**(33): 24–5.

Donabedian A (1988). Quality assessment and assurance; unity of purpose, diversity of means. *Inquiry* **25**: 173–92.

Downie R, Telfer E (1980). *Caring and Curing*. London: Methuen.

Doyle D, ed. (1984). *Palliative Care: The management of advanced illness*. London: Croom Helm.

Doyle D (1987). Orienteering: education and training in palliative care. *Journal of Palliative Care* **2**(2): 5–7.

Doyle D (1991). Palliative care education and training in the United Kingdom: a review. *Death Studies* **15**(1): 95–103.

Dracup KA, Breu CS (1978). Using nursing research findings to meet the needs of grieving spouses. *Nursing Research.* **27**: 212 –16.

Dunlop RJ, Hockley JM (1990). *Terminal Care Support Teams: The hospital–hospice interface*. Oxford: Oxford University Press.

Dwyer DJ, Schwartz RH, Fox ML (1992). Decision-making autonomy in nursing. *Journal of Nursing Administration* **22**(2): 17–23.

Elliott J (1991). *Action Research for Educational Change*. Buckingham: Open University Press.

Eve A, Jackson A (1994). Palliative care services – where are we now? *Palliative Care Today* **3**(2): 22–3.

Fallowfield L (1993a). Evaluation of counselling in the National Health Service. *Journal of the Royal Society of Medicine* **86**: 429–30.

Fallowfield L (1993b). Giving sad and bad news. *The Lancet* **341**: 476–8.

Farrar A (1992). How much do they want to know? Communicating with dying patients. *Professional Nurse* **7**: 606–9.

Farrell W (1993). Differing approaches to training and practice in counselling. *Journal of the Royal Society of Medicine* **86**: 424–5.

Faulkner, A. (1988). The need for education. *Nursing (London): The Journal of Clinical Practice, Education and Management* **3**: 1014–16.

Faulkner A, Maguire P (1988). The need for support. *Nursing (London): The Journal of Clinical Practice, Education and Management* **3**: 1010–12.

Faulkner A, Webb P, Maguire P (1991). Communication and counselling skills: educating health professionals working in cancer and palliative care. *Patient Education and Counselling* **18**(1): 3–7.

Field D (1984). We didn't want him to die on his own . . . nurses' accounts of nursing dying patients. *Journal of Advanced Nursing* **9**(1): 59–70.

Field D, Kitson C (1986). The practical reality. *Nursing Times* March 19: 33–4.

Firth H, McKeown P, McIntee J, Britton O (1987). Professional depression, burnout and personality in long-stay nursing. *International Journal of Nursing Studies* **24**: 227–37.

Fisher M (1988). Hospice nursing. *Nursing (London): The Journal of Clinical Practice, Education and Management* **3**(32): 8–10.

Folkman S (1984). Personal control and stress and coping processes: A theoretical analysis. *Journal of Personality and Social Psychology* **46**: 839–52.

Folkman S, Lazarus R (1980). An analysis of coping in a middle-aged community sample. *Journal of Health and Social Behaviour* **21**: 219–39.

Ford G (1994). Definition and prospects. *Palliative Care Today* **3**(2): 21.

Franks A, Ahmedzai S (1995). Current and future research in palliative care. *Palliative Care Today* **4**(1): 13–14.

Fraser M (1988). The assessment of interprofessional relationships in nursing within a management syllabus in a nursing degree course. *Nurse Education Today* **8**: 273–7.

Gallego A (1987). Evaluation in nursing education. In: *Nursing Education: Research and development*, Davies B, ed. Buckingham: Croom Helm, pp. 205–212.

Garvey A, Manley K (1992). Understanding quality. *Nursing Standard (RCN Nursing Update)* **6**(52): 3–8.

Gibson C (1995). Standard setting in Southampton. *DQI Network News* (1): 7.

Gibson CM (1991). A concept analysis of empowerment. *Journal of Advanced Nursing* **16**: 354–61.

Glaser B, Strauss A (1965). *Awareness of Dying*. Chicago, IL: Aldine.

Glaser B, Strauss A (1967). *The Discovery of Grounded Theory*. Chicago, IL: Aldine.

Goodwin LD, Goodwin WL (1984). Qualitative vs quantitative research or qualitative and quantitative research? *Nursing Research* **33**: 378–80.

Greater Glasgow Health Board (1995). GGHB deaths in 1994: Cancer and others by place of death. Glasgow, Greater Glasgow Health Board, Department of Public Health.

Greenwood J (1984). Nursing research: a position paper. *Journal of Advanced Nursing* **9**: 77–82.

Greenwood J (1994). Action research; a few details, a caution and something new. *Journal of Advanced Nursing* **20**: 13–18.

Gregory D, English J (1994). The myth of control: suffering in palliative care. *Journal of Palliative Care* **10**(2): 18–22.

Guba E, Lincoln Y (1989). *Fourth Generation Evaluation.* Thousand Oaks, CA: Sage Publications.

Guba E, Lincoln Y (1994). Competing paradigms in qualitative research. In: *Handbook of Qualitative Research*, Denzin N, Lincoln Y, eds. Thousand Oaks, CA: Sage Publications Inc., Chapter 6.

Hagerman Z, Tiffany C (1994). Evaluation of two planned change theories. *Nursing Management* **25**(4): 57–60, 62.

Hampe SO (1975). Needs of grieving spouses in a hospital setting. *Nursing Research* **24**: 113–21.

Hanson E (1994) *The Cancer Nurse's Perspective.* Lancaster: Quay Publishing.

Hanson SO (1994). Issues concerning the familiarity of researchers with the research setting. *Journal of Advanced Nursing* **20**: 940–2.

Harper B, Fulton C (1977). Death: Coping mechanisms of the health professional. *Hospice Nursing (London): The Journal of Clinical Practice, Education and Management* **3**(32): 8–10.

Harris C (1990). The disadvantaged dying. *Nursing Times* **86**(22): 26–9.

Harris J (1995). Personal experience: A heartbreaking lesson. *Nursing Times* **91**(42): 48–9.

Hart E, Bond M (1995). Developing action research in nursing. *Nurse Researcher* **2**(3): 4–13.

Harvey G (1988a). More tools for the job. *Nursing Times* **84**(28): 33–4.

Harvey G (1988b). Raising the standards: The right tools for the job. *Nursing Times* **84**(26): 47–50.

Harvey G (1994). *DYSSY Tutorial Package.* Oxford: National Institute for Nursing.

Health Service Commissioner for England, Scotland and Wales (1995). *Third Report for Session 1994–95; Annual Report for 1994–95.* London: HMSO.

Hek G (1995). Sampling techniques in research. *Journal of Community Nursing* **9**(3): 4–6.

Hempel S (1988). No place to lose a loved one. *Nursing Times* **84**(35): 16–17.

Herth K (1990). Fostering hope in terminally ill people. *Journal of Advanced Nursing* **15**: 1250–9.

Herth K (1993). Hope in the family caregiver of terminally ill people. *Journal of Advanced Nursing* **18**: 538–48.

Higginson I (1993). Palliative care: A review of past changes and future trends. *Journal of Public Health Medicine* **15**(1): 3–8.

Higginson I, Wade A, McCarty M (1990). Palliative care: Views of patients and their families. *British Medical Journal* **301**: 277–81.

Hinds C (1985). The needs of families who care for patients with cancer at home – are we meeting them? *Journal of Advanced Nursing* **10**: 575–81.

Hinds P (1989). Survey of graduate programs in cancer nursing. *Oncology Nursing Forum* **16**: 881–7.

Hingley P (1984). The humane face of nursing . . . stress and the nurse manager. *Nursing Mirror* **159**(21): 19–22.

Hingley P, Harris P (1986a). Stress: Burn-out at senior level. *Nursing Times* **82**(31): 28–9.

Hingley P, Harris P (1986b). Stress: Lowering the tension. *Nursing Times* **82**(32): 52–3.

Hinton J (1981). Sharing or withholding information of dying between husband and wife. *Journal of Psychosomatic Research* **25**: 337–43.

Hiscox C (1991). Stress and its management. *Nursing Standard* **5**(21): 36–40.

Hockley J (1989). Caring for the dying in acute hospitals. *Nursing Times* **85**(39): 47–50.

Hockley JM, Dunlop R, Davies RJ (1988). Survey of distressing symptoms in dying patients and their families in hospital and the response to a symptom control team. *British Medical Journal* **296**: 1715–17.

Hodson P (1990). Whose death is it anyway? *The Observer*, 11th March 1990. In: Hunt G (1991) The truth about terminal cancer. *Nursing (Oxford)* **4**(40): 9–11.

Holden RJ (1991). Responsibility and autonomous nursing practice. *Journal of Advanced Nursing* **16**: 398.

Holmes T, Rahe R (1967). The social readjustment and rating scale. *Journal of Psychosomatic Research* **11**: 213–18.

House E (1993). *Professional Evaluation: Social impact and political consequences*. London: Sage.

Houston S, Kendall J (1992). Psychosocial implications of lung cancer. *Nursing Clinics of North America* **27**: 681–90.

Hull M (1992). Coping strategies of family caregivers in hospice homecare. *Oncology Nursing Forum* **19**: 1179–87.

Hull MM (1989a). A family experience: hospice supported home care of a dying relative, Unpublished thesis, University of Rochester.

Hull, MM (1989b). Family needs and supportive nursing behaviours during terminal cancer: A review. *Oncology Nurses Forum* **16**: 787–92.

Hull MM (1990). Sources of stress for hospice caregiving families. *Hospice Journal* **6**(2): 29–54.

Hunt M (1987). The process of translating research findings into nursing practice. *Journal of Advanced Nursing* **12**: 101–10.

Hunt M (1991a). The identification and provision of care for the terminally ill at home by family members. *Sociology of Health and Illness* **13**: 375–95.

Hunt M (1991b). The truth about terminal cancer. *Nursing (Oxford)* **4**(40): 9–11.

Hurtig WA, Stewin L (1990). The effect of death education and experience on nursing students' attitude towards death. *Journal of Advanced Nursing* **15**: 29–34.

Hyde A (1988). Teaching staff to cope with bereavement. *Health Manpower Management* September: 8.

Iles PA, Auluck R (1990). From organizational to interorganizational development in nursing practice: improving the effectiveness of interdisciplinary teamwork and interagency collaboration. *Journal of Advanced Nursing* **15**: 50–8.

Ingleton C, Faulkner A (1993). Audit in palliative care; a senior nurse perspective. *Nursing Standard* **7**(41): 8–9.

International Dictionary in Physics (1961). In: Bailley R, Clarke M (1989) *Stress and Coping in Nursing*. London: Chapman & Hall.

Jackson A (1995). Source of knowledge. *Nursing Times* **91**(14): 55–7.

Janes J (1992). Facing that final journey. *Nursing Standard* **7**(10): 52–3.

Janis IL (1983). Stress inoculation in health care; theory and research. In: *Stress Reduction and Reduction*, Meichenbaum ME, ed. New York: Plenum Press.

Johnson IS, Cockburn M, Pegler J (1988). The Marie Curie/St Luke's relative support scheme: a home care service for relatives of the terminally ill. *Journal of Advanced Nursing* **13**: 566–70.

Jones A (1991). Actors in an emotional drama: inter-related grief in terminal care. *Professional Nurse* **6**: 598–600, 602–3.

Joni R (1995). Why do qualitative research? *British Medical Journal* **311**: 2.

Kelsey S (1992). Can we care to the end? *Professional Nurse* January: 216–6, 236.

Kestenbaum R (1979). Healthy dying – a paradoxical quest continues. *Journal of Social Issues* **35**(185).

Kirschling JM (1986). The experience of terminal illness on adult family members. Special Issue: Nursing in hospice and terminal care: Research and practice. *Hospice Journal* **2**(1): 121–39.

Kitson A (1986). Quality assurance – The methods of measuring quality. *Nursing Times* August 27: 32–4.

Kitson A (1993). Accountability for quality. *Nursing Standard* **8**(1): 4–6.

Klagsbrun S (1994). Patient, family, and staff suffering. *Journal of Palliative Care* **10**(2): 14–17.

Knight M (1981). A silent conspiracy: coping with dying cancer patients on an acute surgical ward. *Journal of Advanced Nursing* **6**: 221–9.

Kobasa S (1979). Stressful life events; personality and health; an inquiry into hardiness. in Strumpfer DJW (1990). Salutogenesis: A new paradigm. *South African Journal of Psychology* **24**: 265–76.

Koch T (1992). A review of nursing quality assurance. *Journal of Advanced Nursing* **17**: 795.

Kristjanson L (1986). Indicators of quality of family care from a family perspective. *Journal of Palliative Care* **1**(2): 8–17.

Kristjanson LJ (1989). Quality of terminal care: salient indicators identified by families. *Journal of Palliative Care* **5**(1): 21–30.

Kristjanson LJ (1993). Validity and reliability testing of the Famcare Scale – measuring family satisfaction with advanced cancer care. *Social Science & Medicine* **36**(5): 693–701.

Kristjanson L, Ashcroft T (1994). The family's cancer journey: a literature review. *Cancer Nursing* **17**(1): 1–17.

Kristjanson LJ, Scanlan JM (1989). Assessment of continuing nursing education needs: a literature review. *Journal of Continuing Education in Nursing* **20**: 118–23.

Kvale S (1983). The qualitative research interview: A phenomenological and hermeneutical mode of understanding. *Journal of Phenomenological Psychology* **14**: 171–96.

Lamb G, Huttlinger K (1991). Reflexivity in nursing research. *Western Journal of Nursing Research* **11**: 765–72.

Lang N, Wessel Krejci J (1991). Standards and holism: A reframing. *Holistic Nursing Practice* **5**(3): 14–21.

Larsson G, Kallenberg K, Setterlind S, Starrin B (1994). Health and loss of a family member; Impact on sense of coherence. *International Journal of Health Sciences* **5**(1): 5–11.

Lathlean J, Farnish S (1984). *The Ward Sister Training Project: An evaluation of a training scheme.* Report. Nursing Education Research Unit, Department of Nursing, Kings College London.

Lattimer V (1991). Evaluating teaching effectiveness. In: *Curriculum Planning in Nurse Education*, Pendleton S, Myles, A, eds. London: Edward Arnold, pp. 187–9.

Lazarus R (1985). The psychology of stress and coping – urban people of Israel. *Issues in Mental Health Nursing* **7**: 399–418.

Lazarus R, Folkman S (1984). *Stress, Appraisal and Coping*. New York: Springer Verlag.

Lazarus RS (1976). *Patterns of Adjustment*. New York: McGraw-Hill.

Leefarr V, Cutler M (1994). Stress. In: *Nursing Practice Hospital and Home. The adult*, Alexander M, Fawcet J, Runciman P, eds. Edinburgh: Churchill Livingstone, 575–96.

Leininger M (1984). Ethnography and ethnonursing; models and modes of qualitative analysis. In: *Qualitative Research Methods in Nursing*, Leininger M, ed. Orlando, FL: Grune & Stratton Inc., pp. 48–57.

Leonard V (1989). A Heideggerian phenomenologic perspective on the concept of the person. *Advances in Nursing Science* **11**(4): 40–55.

Leonard V (1994). A Heideggerian phenomenological perspective on the concept of person. *Interpretive Phenomenology: Embodiment caring and ethics in health and illness*, Benner P, ed. Thousand Oaks, CA: Sage Publications Inc., pp. 43–63.

Lewandowski W, Jones SL (1988). The family with cancer: Nursing interventions throughout the course of living with cancer. *Cancer Nursing* **11**: 313–21.

Lewin K (1951). *Field Theory in Social Sciences: Selected theoretical papers*. New York: Harper & Row.

Lewis FM (1986). The impact of cancer on the family: A critical analysis of the research literature. *Patient Education and Counselling* **8**: 279–89.

Lugton J (1987). *Communicating with Dying People and Their Relatives*. London: Austen Cornish Publishers Ltd, in association with the Lisa Sainsbury Foundation.

Lugton J (1989a). Relatives – Communicating in the hospice. *Nursing Times*. **85**(16): 28–30.

Lugton J (1989b). Relatives – Identifying anxieties. *Nursing Times* **85**(17): 50–1.

Luker K (1981). An overview of evaluation research in nursing. *Journal of Advanced Nursing* (6): 87–93.

Lutjens L, Tiffany C (1994). Evaluating planned change theories. *Nursing Management* **25**(3): 54–7.

Lyons GJ (1988). Bereavement and death education – a survey of nurses' views. *Nurse Education Today* **8**: 168–72.

McGhee M (1994). The impact of grief. *Update* June: 9089–10.

McGrath A, Reid N, Boore JRP (1989). Occupational stress in nursing. *International Journal of Nursing Studies* **26**: 343–58.

McHaffie H (1992). Coping: an essential element in nursing. *Journal of Advanced Nursing* **17**: 933–40.

Mackenzie A (1994). Evaluating ethnography: considerations for analysis. *Journal of Advanced Nursing* **19**: 774–81.

Mackenzie J (1992). Clinical standards – Dilemmas in setting quality standards. *Nursing Standard* **6**(29): 37–9.

McWhan K (1991). Caring for dying patients in acute hospital wards: a review. *Nursing Practice* **5**(1): 25–8.

Maguire P (1985a). Barriers to psychological care of the dying. *British Medical Journal* **291**: 1711–3.

Maguire P (1985b). Consequences of poor communication between nurses and patients. *Nursing (Oxford)* **2**: 1115–16, 1118.

Maguire P (1988). The stress of communicating with seriously ill patients. *Nursing (London): The Journal of Clinical Practice, Education and Management* **3**(32): 25–7.

Maguire P, Faulkner A (1988). Improve the counselling skills of doctors and nurses in cancer care. *British Medical Journal* **297**: 847–9.

Marks M (1992). Palliative care. *Nursing Standard (RCN Nursing Update)* **6**(33): 9–14.

Marsland D, Gissane C (1992). Nursing evaluation: purposes achievements and opportunities. *International Journal of Nursing Studies* **29**: 231–6.

Maslin-Prothero S (1992). Women nursing and caring; the issues. *Nursing Standard* **7**(7): 25–8.

Matson CA (1988). Families with a terminally ill member: A grounded theory of family relationships. *American Journal of Hospital Care* **5**(4): 38–41.

Mayer D (1986). Cancer patients' and families' perceptions of nurse caring behaviors. *Topics in Clinical Nursing* **8**(2): 63–9.

Mays N, Pope C (1995). Rigour and qualitative research. *British Medical Journal* **311**: 109–12.

Melia KM (1982). 'Tell it as it is' – qualitative methodology and nursing research: understanding the student nurse's world. *Journal of Advanced Nursing* **7**: 327–35.

Methot D, Caesar J, Duquette DM (1992). Empowering staff nurses through quality assurance. *Journal of Nursing Care Quality* **6**(2): 9–14.

Meyer J (1993). New paradigm research in practice. *Journal of Advanced Nursing* **18**: 1066–72.

Miles MB, Huberman MA (1984). Drawing valid meaning from qualitative data: Towards a shared craft. *Educational Researcher* **13**: 20–30.

Mitchell A (1987). A conspiracy of silence. *Senior Nurse* **7**(2): 20–1.

Monet A, Lazarus R (1985). *Stress and coping: An anthology*. New York: Columbia University Press.

Morris E (1988). A pain of separation – how can nurses best assist the dying and the bereaved? *Nursing Times* **84**(42): 54–6.

Moynihan C (1993). A history of counselling. *Journal of the Royal Society of Medicine* **86**: 421–3.

Muir C, Harvey J (1994). Scottish cancer statistics ll. *Newsletter of the Scottish Cancer Therapy Network* (3): 11–14.

Nash A (1989). A terminal case? Burnout in palliative care. *The Professional Nurse* 443–4.

Nganasurian W (1992). Stress and its management through research. *Senior Nurse* **12**(4): 40–3.

Nixon P (1993). The broken heart – counteraction by SABRES. *Journal of the Royal Society of Medicine* **86**: 468–71.

Norbeck J (1986). Perceived job stress, job satisfaction and psychological symptoms in critical care nursing. *Research in Nursing and Health* **8**: 252–9.

Northouse P, Northouse L (1987). Communication and cancer: issues confronting patients health professionals and family members. *Journal of Psychosocial Oncology* **5**: 17–46.

Nugent LS (1988). The social support requirements of family caregivers of terminal cancer patients. *Canadian Journal of Nursing Research* **20**(3): 45–58.

Oberle K, Davies B (1992). Support and caring : Exploring the concepts. *Oncology Nursing Forum* **17**: 763–7.

Oberle K, Davies B (1993). An exploration of nursing disillusionment. *The Canadian Journal of Nursing Research* **25**(1): 67–75.

Oberst M, Thomas S, Ward SE (1989). Caregiving demands and appraisal of stress among family caregivers. *Cancer Nursing* **12**: 209–15.

Oiler Boyd C (1993). Towards a nursing practice research method. *Advances in Nursing Science* **16**(2): 9–15.

Owen D (1989). Nurses' perspectives on the meaning of hope in patients with cancer: a qualitative study. *Oncology Nursing Forum* **16**(1): 75–9.

Padilla R (1993). *HyperQual2*. Chandler, AZ: the author.

Parkes CM (1978). Home or hospital? – Terminal care as seen by surviving spouses. *Journal of the Royal College of General Practitioners* **28**: 19–30.

Parkes CM (1988). Not always. Special Issue: Controversies in palliative care: A thematic issue. *Journal of Palliative Care* **4**(1–2): 50–2.

Parlett M, Hamilton D (1972). Evaluation as illumination. In: *Introduction to Illuminative Evaluation: Studies in higher education*, Parlett M, Dearden G, eds. Cardiff-By-The-Sea, CA: Soundings Press.

Parse R, ed. (1995). Research with the human becoming theory. *Illuminations: The human becoming theory in practice and research*. New York: National League for Nursing Press, Pub. No. 15-2670.

Paulen A (1980). *Standards for Person-centred Caring*. Madison, WI: University Hospital.

Pearlin L, Schooler C (1978). The structure of coping. *Journal of Health and Social Behaviour* **19**: 2–21.

Perakyla A (1991). Hope work in the care of seriously ill patients. *Qualitative Health Research* **1**: 407–33.

Polit D, Hungler B (1991). *Nursing Research: Principles and methods*. Philadelphia: JP Lippincott Co.

Poulton B (1992). Setting standards of care. *Nursing Standard (RCN Nursing Update)* **7**(2): 3–8.

Powers B, Knapp T (1995). *A Dictionary of Nursing Theory and Research*. Thousand Oaks, CA: Sage Publications.

Redfern S, Norman I (1990). Measuring the quality of nursing care; a consideration of different approaches. *Journal of Advanced Nursing* **15**: 1260–71.

Reeder F (1987). The phenomenological movement. *Image: Journal of Nursing Scholarship* **19**: 150–2.

Reeder F (1988). Hermeneutics. In: *Paths to Knowledge: Innovative research methods for nursing*, Sarter B, ed. New York: National League for Nursing, pp. 193–238.

Registrar General for Scotland (1994). *Populations Statistics Branch Report*. Edinburgh: General Register Office for Scotland.

Reinharz S (1983). Phenomenology as a dynamic process. *Phenomenology and Pedagogy* **1**: 77–9.

Rotter JB (1966). Generalized expectancies for internal versus external locus of control. In: Strumpfer DJW (1990). Salutogenesis: A new paradigm. *South African Journal of Psychology* **20**: 265–76.

Royal College of Nursing (1991). *Standards of Care for Cancer Nursing*. Harrow: Scutari Press.

Russell G (1993). The role of denial in clinical practice. *Journal of Advanced Nursing* **18**: 938–40.

Sale D (1988). Raising the standards – down Dorset way. *Nursing Times* **84**(28): 31–2.

Sandelowski M (1986). The problem of rigor in qualitative research. *Advances in Nursing Science* **8**(3): 27–37.

Sandelowski M (1991). Telling stories: narrative approaches in qualitative research. *Image: Journal of Nursing Scholarship* **23**: 161–6.

Sandelowski M (1993a). Theory unmasked: The uses and guises of theory in qualitative research. *Research in Nursing and Health* **16**: 213–18.

Sandelowski M (1993b). Rigor or rigor mortis: the problem of rigor in qualitative work revisited. *Advances in Nursing Science* **16**(2): 1–8.

Sandelowski M, Davis DH, Harris BG (1989). Artful design: writing the proposal for research in the naturalist paradigm. *Research in Nursing and Health* **12**(2): 77–84.

Saunders JM, Valente SM (1994). Nurses' grief. *Cancer Nursing* **17**: 318–25.

Scanlon C (1989). Creating a vision of hope; the challenge of palliative care. *Oncology Nurses Forum* **16**: 189–283.

Schermerhorn J (1981). Guidelines for change in health care organizations. *Health Care Management Review* **6**(3): 9.

Schon D (1987). *Educating the Reflective Practitioner*. San Francisco, CA: Jossey Bass.

Schutz A (1970). *On Phenomenology and Social Relations*. Chicago: University of Chicago Press.

Scottish Office (1991). *The Patient's Charter – A Charter for Health*. Edinburgh: HMSO.

Scottish Partnership Agency for Palliative and Cancer Care (1995). Directory of palliative care services in Scotland 1995. Edinburgh: Scottish Partnership Agency for Palliative and Cancer Care in conjunction with the Health Education Board for Scotland.

Seale C (1991). Communication and awareness about death – a study of a random sample of dying people. *Social Science and Medicine* **32**: 943–52.

Seale C (1992). Community nurses and the care of the dying. *Social Science and Medicine* **34**: 375–82.

Seale C (1993). Changes in death and dying: the past 25 years. *Critical Public Health* **4**(3): 4–11.

Seale CF (1989). What happens in hospices: a review of research evidence. *Social Science and Medicine* **28**: 551–9.

Selye H (1974). *Stress without Distress*. London: Hodder & Stoughton.

Shea T, Kendrick K (1995). 'With velvet gloves': the ethics of collusion. *Palliative Care Today* **4**(1): 9–10.

Simpson K (1989). Understanding mourning. *Nursing Times* **85**(4): 43–5.

Skorupka P, Bohnet N (1982). Primary caregivers' perceptions of nursing behaviors that best meet their needs in a home care hospice setting. *Cancer Nursing* **5**: 371–4.

Smith NA, Ley P, Seale JP, Shaw J (1987). Health beliefs, satisfaction, and compliance. *Patient Education and Counseling* **10**: 279–86.

Steptoe A, Sutcliffe I, Allen B, Coombes C (1991). Satisfaction with communication, medical knowledge, and coping style in patients with metastatic cancer. *Social Science and Medicine* **32**: 627–32.

Stetz KM (1987). Caregiver demands during advanced cancer – the spouses needs. *Cancer Nursing* **10**: 260–8.

Stetz KM, Hanson WK (1992). Alterations in perceptions of caregiving demands in advanced cancer during and after the experience. *Hospice Journal* **8**(3): 21–34.

Stevenson D (1990). The energy crisis of change. *Nursing Practice* **4**(1): 15–17.

Strumpfer D (1990). Salutogenesis: A new paradigm. *South African Journal of Psychology* **20**: 265–76.

Suchman E (1967). *Evaluation Research*. Rochester, NY: Russell Sage Foundation.

Sudnow D (1967). *Passing On: The social organisation of dying*. New York: Prentice Hall.

Sutor J (1993). Can nurses be effective advocates? *Nursing Standard* **17**(7): 30–32.

Swansburg RC (1993). *Introductory Management and Clinical Leadership for Clinical Nurses.* Boston: James & Bartlett Publishers Inc.

Swanson-Kauffman K, Schonwald E (1988). Phenomenology. In: *Paths to Knowledge; Innovative research methods for nursing*, Sarter B, ed. New York: National League for Nurses, pp. 97–105.

Tappen R (1989). *Nursing Leadership and Management: Concepts and practice.* Philadelphia, PA: FA Davis Co.

Tesch R (1990). *Qualitative Research – Analysis, types and software tools.* New York: Falmer Press.

Thorne S (1985). The family cancer experience. *Cancer Nursing* **8**: 285–91.

Thorne S (1991). Methodological orthodoxy in qualitative nursing research; analysis of the issues. *Qualitative Health Research* **1**: 178–99.

Tiffany C, Cheatham A, Doornbos D, Loudermelt L, Momadi GG (1994). Planned change theory; survey of nursing periodical literature. *Nursing Management* **25**(7): 55–9.

Titchen A (1995). Issues of validity in action research. *Nurse Researcher* **2**(3): 38–48.

Titchen A, Binnie A (1993). Research partnerships: collaborative action research in nursing. *Journal of Advanced Nursing* **18**: 858–65.

United Kingdom Central Council (1992). *Code of Professional Conduct for Nurses, Midwives and Health Visitors*, 3rd edn. London: UKCC.

Waddell D (1991) Differentiating impact evaluation from evaluation research: one perspective of implications for continuing nursing education. *The Journal of Continuing Education in Nursing* **22**(6): 254–8.

Wainwright S (1994). Analysing data using grounded theory. *Nurse Researcher* **1**(3): 43–7.

Walters AJ (1994). A hermeneutic study of the concept of 'focusing' in critical care nursing practice. *Nursing Inquiry* **1**: 23–30.

Waterman H (1995). Distinguishing between 'traditional' and action research. *Nurse Researcher* **2**(3): 15–23.

Waterson J (1992). Nursing's feminist tuition. *Nursing Standard* **7**(7): 56.

Watson J (1990). Knowledge about care and caring: state of the art and future developments. *Human Caring: A public agenda.* American Nurses' Association Publications, American Academy of Nursing no. G-177: 41-8 (Pamphlet).

Watson MJ (1988). New dimensions of human caring theory. *Nursing Science Quarterly* **1**: 175–81.

Weatherall D (1994). The inhumanity of medicine; time to stop and think (editorial). *British Medical Journal* **309**: 1671.

Webb C (1989). Action research: philosophy, methods and personal experiences. *Journal of Advanced Nursing* **14**: 403–10.

Webber J (1993). A specialised role in the health care setting. *Nursing Standard* **7**(19): 52–3.

Weisman A (1979). *Coping with Cancer.* New York: McGraw Hill.

Wilkinson S (1991). Factors which influence how nurses communicate with cancer patients. *Journal of Advanced Nursing* **16** : 677–88.

Wilkinson S (1992). Good communication in cancer nursing. *Nursing Standard* **7**(9): 35–9.

Wilson HS, Hutchieson S (1991). Triangulation of qualitative methods: Heideggerian Hermeneutics and grounded theory. *Qualitative Health Research* **1**: 263–76.

Wilson S, Morse JM (1991). Living with a wife undergoing chemotherapy. *Image: Journal of Nursing Scholarship* **23**(2): 78–84.

Winters J (1992). Mentorship for everyone. *Nursing Standard* **7**(7): 44–5.

Woods NF, Lewis MF, Ellison ES (1989). Living with cancer: family experience. *Cancer Nursing* **12**(1): 28–33.

Worden J (1983). *Grief Counselling and Grief Therapy*. London: Tavistock.

World Health Organization (1990). *Cancer Pain Relief and Palliative Care*. Geneva: WHO Expert Committee; Technical Report. Series No. 804.

Wright A, Cousins J, Upward J (1988). *Matters of Death and Life: a study of bereavement support in NHS hospitals in England*. King Edwards Hospital Fund for London.

Wright S (1989). *Changing Nursing Practice*. London: Edward Arnold.

Wros P (1993). *Behind the Curtain: Nursing care of dying patients in critical care*. OR: Oregon Health Science University School of Nursing.

Wros PL (1994). The ethical context of nursing care of dying patients in critical care. In: *Interpretive Phenomenology: Embodiment, caring and ethics in health and illness*, Benner P, ed. Thousand Oaks, CA: Sage Publications, pp. 255–77.

Wrubel J, Benner P, Lazarus RS (1981). Social competence from the perspective of stress and coping. In: *Social Competence*, Wine J, Smye M, eds. New York: Guilford Press, pp. 61–99.

Youll JW (1989). The bridge beyond: strengthening nursing practice in attitudes towards death, dying, and the terminally ill, and helping the spouses of critically ill patients. *Intensive Care Nursing* **5**(2): 88–9.

Index

Page numbers in *italic* refer to tables

257